METABOLIC RESET DIET FOR WOMEN

Ignite Your Metabolism, Transform Your Body:
Unleash the Power of the Metabolic Reset Diet.

MICHELLE O. LEWIS

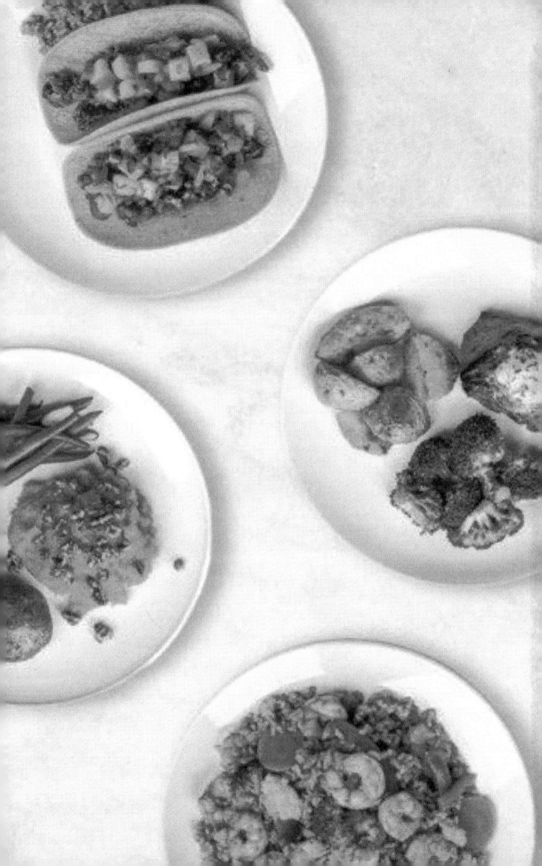

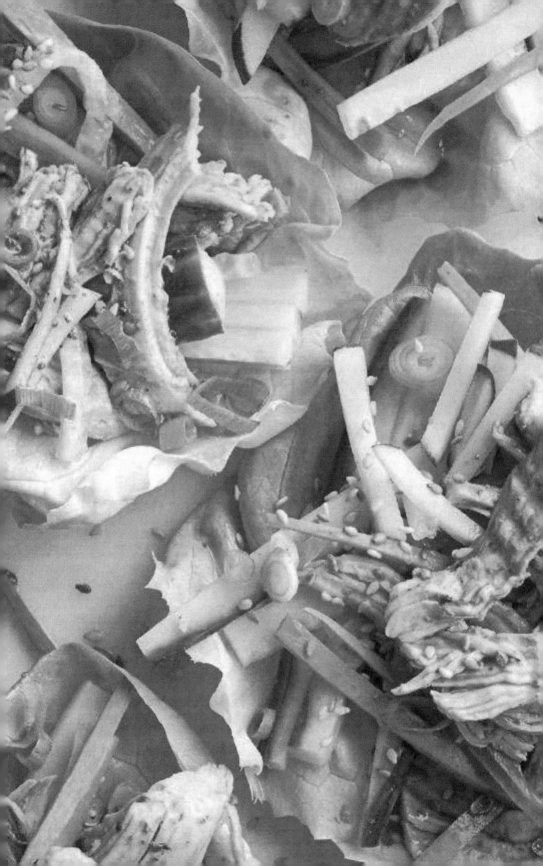

Printed in the United States of America.

First Edition: January 2024

TABLE OF CONTENT

INTRODUCTION 2

Overview of the Metabolic Reset Diet: Nurturing Your Body From Within 7

The Importance of Metabolism for Women's Health and Weight Management 10

Addressing Common Concerns and Desires Related to Metabolism 13

Chapter 1: 17

Understanding Metabolism 17

What Is Metabolism and How It Works: Decoding the Body's Engine 17

Factors that Influence Metabolism in Women: Navigating the Female Metabolic Landscape 19

Impact of Age, Genetics, and Lifestyle on Metabolism 21

Common Misconceptions About Metabolism: Dispelling Myths and Fostering Understanding 23

Chapter 2: 25

Hormonal Balance and Metabolism 25

The Connection Between Hormones and Metabolism: Harmonizing Body Functions 25

Hormonal Imbalances and their Impact on Weight Management 27

Strategies to Support Hormonal Balance for Optimal Metabolism: Nurturing Hormonal Harmony 29

Addressing Specific Hormonal Concerns (e.g., PCOS, Menopause) 31

Chapter 3:..**34**

The Metabolic Reset Diet Principles **34**

Overview of the Metabolic Reset Diet Approach: A Holistic Blueprint for Wellness..**34**

Balancing Macronutrients for Metabolic Optimization..........**36**

Understanding Calorie Intake and Expenditure.....................**38**

Importance of Nutrient-Dense Foods and Portion Control: Crafting A Balanced Plate **40**

Chapter 4:..**43**

Resetting Your Metabolism: Phase 1 ....**43**

Specific Guidelines for Phase 1: Navigating Food Choices and Meal Planning **45**

Strategies to Support Detoxification and Elimination of Toxins: Cleansing for Metabolic Clarity.............................**47**

Sample Meal Plans and Recipes for Phase 1: Practical Tools for Success **49**

14-Day Sample Meal Plan: Metabolic Reset Diet **49**

Recipes for Phase 1: **57**

1. Grilled Chicken and Quinoa Salad with Lemon-Tahini Dressing:..57

2. Detoxifying Green Smoothie Bowl: 58

3. Baked Salmon with Dill and Asparagus:...........................59

4. Quinoa and Black Bean Stuffed Bell Peppers:....................60

5. Lemon Garlic Shrimp Stir-Fry with Broccoli and Cauliflower Rice: 61

6. Greek Yogurt Parfait with Berries and Almond Granola: ...62

7. Avocado and Chickpea Lettuce Wraps: 62

8. Zucchini Noodles with Pesto and Grilled Chicken:.............63

9. Detoxifying Cucumber and Mint Infused Water:.................64

10. Berry and Spinach Salad with Almond-Crusted Salmon:..64

11. Grilled Lemon Herb Salmon:..65

12. Detox Lentil Soup:...66

13. Baked Lemon Herb Chicken: 67

14. Detoxifying Green Detoxifying Green Salad:...................68

15. Detoxifying Turmeric Ginger Smoothie: 69

16. Sweet Potato and Kale Hash with Poached Eggs:..........70

17. Cauliflower and Broccoli Detox Soup:..............................71

18. Quinoa and Vegetable Stir-Fry: 72

19. Turmeric and Garlic Baked Chicken Thighs: 73

20. Chia Seed Pudding with Mixed Berries: 74

Chapter 5:...**75**

Resetting Your Metabolism: Phase 2 ....**75**

Transitioning from Phase 1 to Phase 2 of the Metabolic Reset Diet...**75**

Adjusting Macronutrient Ratios and Calorie Intake...............**77**

Incorporating Exercise and Physical Activity for Metabolic Enhancement..**78**

Sample Meal Plans and Recipes for Phase 2 ....**79**

Sample Meal Plan: 79

Recipes For Phase 2...**88**

Quinoa Salad with Roasted Vegetables and Grilled Chicken...88

Turkey and Avocado Wrap 89

1. Grilled Salmon and Quinoa Power Bowl: 90

2. Mediterranean Chickpea and Vegetable Stir-Fry:............90

3. Quinoa and Kale Stuffed Bell Peppers: 91

4. Lemon Herb Chicken with Asparagus and Brown Rice: 92

5. Spinach and Feta Turkey Burgers:................................92

6. Roasted Vegetable and Quinoa Salad: 93

7. Tofu and Vegetable Coconut Curry: 94

8. Shrimp and Vegetable Stir-Fry with Cauliflower Rice: 94

9. Avocado and Quinoa Stuffed Portobello Mushrooms:......95

10. Teriyaki Chicken and Broccoli Brown Rice Bowl: 96

11. Veggie Egg Muffins: 97

12. Greek Yogurt Parfait:..98

13. Baked Salmon with Lemon-Dill Sauce: 98

14. Turkey and Vegetable Stir-Fry:................................99

15. Grilled Lemon Herb Chicken: 100

16. Baked Cod with Roasted Vegetables:...................... 101

17. Quinoa and Black Bean Salad:............................. 102

Chapter 6:...**105**

Maintaining a Healthy Metabolism **105**

Strategies for Long-Term Sustainability and Maintenance..**105**

Building Healthy Habits and A Balanced Lifestyle **107**

Tips for Overcoming Plateaus and Challenges.....................**109**

Mindset and Motivation for Sustained Success.....................**111**

Chapter 7:...**113**

Beyond the Diet: Supporting Overall Health.........................**113**

Importance of Holistic Health Beyond Just Metabolism......**113**

Addressing Digestive Health and Gut Microbiome **115**

Managing Stress and Sleep for Optimal Metabolism **117**

Supplements and Additional Support for Women's Health .**119**

Conclusion: 121

Recap Of Key Concepts and Takeaways From The Metabolic Reset Diet...121

Encouragement And Motivation for Readers to Embark on Their Metabolic Reset Journey 124

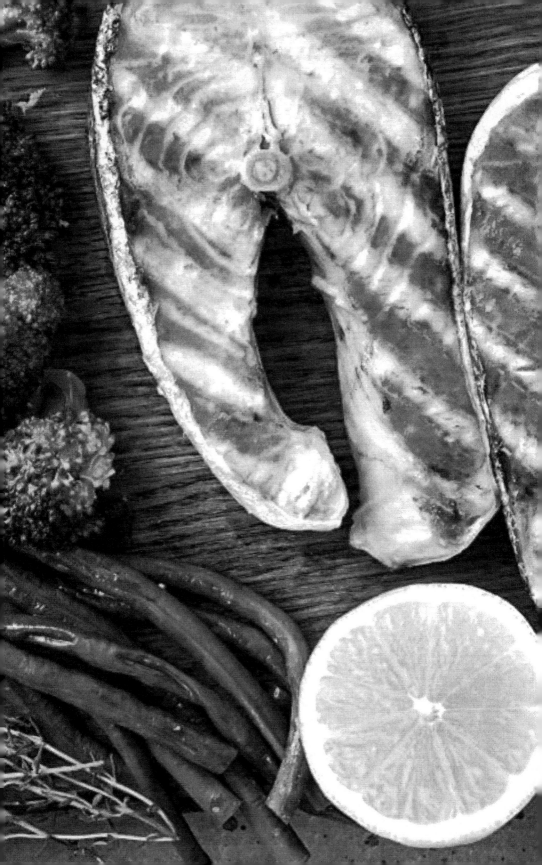

INTRODUCTION

Welcome to a transformative journey towards optimal health and vitality. Imagine a life where your metabolism is a powerful force, working in harmony with your body to achieve your desired weight and overall well-being. This is the promise of the metabolic reset diet for women.

In a world filled with fad diets and quick fixes, it's essential to understand the true importance of metabolism for women's health and weight management. Your metabolism is like a symphony, with each instrument playing a vital role in the harmony of your body's functions. When your metabolism is in sync, you feel energized, vibrant, and confident in your own skin.

But all too often, women find themselves battling against their metabolism, struggling to shed unwanted pounds or feeling trapped in a cycle of fatigue and frustration. It's time to break free from these limitations and unlock the secrets to optimizing your metabolism.

Picture this: You wake up in the morning feeling refreshed and ready to conquer the day. Your body is a well-oiled machine, efficiently converting food into energy and effortlessly maintaining your ideal weight. With each passing day, you notice a renewed sense of vitality and a newfound confidence radiating from within.

Now, let's address the common concerns and desires that women have when it comes to their metabolism. Perhaps you've tried countless diets, only to be left feeling deprived and defeated. You may have experienced the frustration of hitting a weight loss plateau or struggling with hormonal imbalances that seem to sabotage your efforts. These challenges are all too familiar, but they don't have to define your journey.

Through the metabolic reset diet, we will delve deep into the intricacies of your metabolism, unraveling the mysteries that have held you back. We will address the specific concerns that women face, from hormonal balance to stubborn weight gain, and provide you with practical solutions that are rooted in science and tailored to your unique needs.

Imagine feeling empowered as you navigate the aisles of the grocery store, confidently selecting foods that nourish your body and fuel your metabolism. Picture yourself enjoying delicious meals that not only satisfy your taste buds but also support your journey towards optimal health. This is the power of the metabolic reset diet.

Together, we will embark on a journey of self-discovery and transformation. We will explore the intricate dance between your metabolism and overall well-being, uncovering the secrets that will unlock your full potential.

Get ready to rewrite your story and embrace a life where your metabolism becomes your greatest ally.

Are you ready to embark on this remarkable adventure? Let's dive into the metabolic reset diet and unlock the vibrant, energetic, and confident woman within you.

Embarking on a journey toward optimal health and sustainable weight management is a profound undertaking, and the key to success often lies in understanding and harnessing the power of metabolism. In this introductory chapter, we delve into the concept of the Metabolic Reset Diet for Women, exploring its foundations, significance, and the transformative impact it can have on women's overall well-being.

Understanding Metabolic Reset: A Holistic Approach to Wellness

The Metabolic Reset Diet is not just another fad; it's a comprehensive and holistic approach designed specifically for women. It goes beyond traditional dieting by addressing the intricacies of the body's metabolism. This reset is not about restrictive eating or short-term solutions; instead, it aims to restore balance, optimize energy expenditure, and promote sustainable weight management.

The journey begins with a profound shift in perspective—a realization that our bodies are dynamic, adaptable systems that respond to the way we nourish and care for them. The Metabolic Reset Diet embraces this understanding, guiding women toward a lifestyle that aligns with their unique metabolic needs.

Embarking on the Metabolic Reset Journey: What to Expect

Before we delve into the intricacies of metabolic health and weight management, it's essential to set realistic expectations for the journey ahead. The Metabolic Reset Diet is not a quick fix or a one-size-fits-all solution. Instead, it's a personalized exploration, a commitment to understanding and nourishing your body in a way that promotes lasting change.

Throughout this guide, we'll explore the science behind metabolism, the factors influencing women's metabolic health, and practical strategies to implement a successful reset. From nutrition tips and lifestyle adjustments to mindset shifts, each aspect contributes to a comprehensive reset tailored to the unique needs of women.

Why Metabolic Health Matters: Beyond Weight Loss

Metabolic health is a cornerstone of overall well-being for women. It influences not only weight management but also energy levels, mood, hormonal balance, and longevity. As we age or face life changes such as pregnancy or menopause, our metabolism undergoes shifts that can impact various aspects of our health.

The Metabolic Reset Diet acknowledges the interconnected nature of these factors, offering a roadmap to rejuvenate metabolism for improved vitality and resilience. By prioritizing metabolic health, women can achieve a balanced and sustainable approach to weight management, ensuring that their bodies function optimally in every stage of life.

Overview of the Metabolic Reset Diet: Nurturing Your Body from Within

In this section, we provide a comprehensive overview of the Metabolic Reset Diet, outlining its fundamental principles and explaining how it differs from conventional diets. From understanding the role of macronutrients to exploring the importance of meal timing, each aspect contributes to a well-rounded approach to metabolic reset.

Foundations of the Metabolic Reset Diet

At the heart of the Metabolic Reset Diet lies a foundation built on science, balance, and sustainability. Unlike restrictive diets that focus solely on calorie reduction, this approach emphasizes the quality of nutrients, acknowledging that our bodies require a diverse range of vitamins, minerals, and macronutrients for optimal function.

We delve into the significance of whole, nutrient-dense foods and their role in supporting metabolism. From lean proteins and complex carbohydrates to healthy fats and micronutrient-rich vegetables, each component plays a crucial role in nourishing the body and promoting metabolic efficiency.

The Role of Macronutrients in Metabolic Optimization

Understanding the role of macronutrients—proteins, carbohydrates, and fats—is pivotal in crafting a diet that supports metabolic reset. Proteins, often hailed as the building blocks of the body, contribute to muscle health and satiety. Carbohydrates, when chosen wisely, provide sustainable energy, while healthy fats support hormone production and absorption of fat-soluble vitamins.

This section explores the optimal balance of macronutrients tailored to women's metabolic needs. It dispels common misconceptions and offers practical insights into creating meals that fuel the body while promoting a healthy weight.

Meal Timing and Frequency: A Strategic Approach

Beyond the composition of meals, the Metabolic Reset Diet recognizes the importance of meal timing and frequency. We delve into the science of circadian rhythms and how aligning eating patterns with the body's natural cycles can enhance metabolic function.

The discussion extends to the concept of intermittent fasting, exploring its potential benefits for women's metabolic health. By adopting a strategic approach to meal timing, individuals can optimize energy utilization, support digestion, and regulate hormonal balance.

Balancing Hormones for Metabolic Harmony

Hormones play a pivotal role in women's metabolic health, influencing everything from appetite to fat storage. The Metabolic Reset Diet addresses the delicate balance of hormones, offering insights into nutrition and lifestyle choices that promote hormonal harmony.

From cortisol management to supporting thyroid function, this section provides practical tips for women to nurture their endocrine system. By understanding the intricate interplay of hormones, individuals can make informed choices that contribute to a balanced and thriving metabolism.

The Importance of Metabolism for Women's Health and Weight Management

Understanding metabolism is central to unlocking the secrets of women's health and effective weight management. In this segment, we delve into the intricacies of metabolism, its role in the female body, and how various factors impact its efficiency.

Metabolism Unveiled: A Comprehensive Overview

Metabolism is often simplified to the notion of burning calories, but its complexity extends far beyond. This section unravels the intricacies of metabolism, explaining how the body converts food into energy, regulates weight, and maintains vital functions.

We explore the distinction between basal metabolic rate (BMR) and total daily energy expenditure (TDEE), shedding light on how these factors influence the calories burned in rest and during physical activity. Understanding this metabolic baseline sets the stage for effective weight management strategies.

Metabolic Factors Unique to Women

Women's metabolic health is influenced by factors unique to their physiology, including hormonal fluctuations, reproductive stages, and genetic predispositions. This segment delves into how hormonal changes during menstruation, pregnancy, and menopause can impact metabolism and weight regulation.

By acknowledging and understanding these nuances, women can tailor their approach to metabolic reset, adapting strategies that align with their specific needs at different life stages. The Metabolic Reset Diet embraces these differences, offering a personalized roadmap for women to achieve optimal metabolic health.

The Impact of Lifestyle on Metabolic Efficiency

While genetics and hormonal factors play a significant role, lifestyle choices also exert a profound influence on metabolic health. From sleep quality and stress management to physical activity and hydration, every aspect of lifestyle contributes to the efficiency of metabolism.

This section explores how adopting healthy habits can positively impact metabolic function. Practical tips for incorporating movement into daily life, managing stress, and prioritizing quality sleep offer women actionable steps toward nurturing their metabolism.

Metabolic Challenges and Solutions

Many women face challenges such as a sluggish metabolism, weight fluctuations, or difficulty losing weight despite efforts to diet and exercise. This part of the chapter addresses common metabolic challenges and provides targeted solutions.

We discuss the impact of yo-yo dieting, the role of muscle mass in metabolism, and the potential pitfalls of overly restrictive diets. By identifying these challenges, women can proactively implement strategies to overcome hurdles and optimize their metabolic potential.

Addressing Common Concerns and Desires Related to Metabolism

In this section, we address prevalent concerns and desires women have related to metabolism. From the desire for sustainable weight loss to concerns about energy levels and hormonal balance, we provide insights and solutions that align with the principles of the Metabolic Reset Diet.

Sustainable Weight Loss: Beyond Quick Fixes

One of the most common desires related to metabolism is achieving sustainable weight loss. However, the Metabolic Reset Diet distinguishes itself from quick fixes and restrictive diets. This part of the chapter emphasizes the importance of adopting a holistic approach that prioritizes long-term health over rapid, unsustainable results.

We explore the science behind gradual and sustainable weight loss, emphasizing the role of metabolism in achieving and maintaining a healthy body weight. By setting realistic goals and implementing gradual lifestyle changes, women can achieve lasting success without compromising their well-being.

Boosting Energy Levels: The Metabolic Reset Solution

Low energy levels are a concern shared by many women, often attributed to factors such as stress, poor sleep, or imbalanced nutrition. This section of the chapter outlines how the Metabolic Reset Diet addresses these concerns by optimizing energy production at the cellular level.

We discuss the role of nutrient-dense foods, strategic meal timing, and the avoidance of energy-draining habits. By aligning nutritional choices with metabolic needs, women can experience sustained energy throughout the day, supporting overall vitality and well-being.

Hormonal Harmony: Nurturing Women's Endocrine Health

Balancing hormones is a key desire for many women seeking to optimize their metabolic health. This part of the chapter delves into the intricate connection between nutrition, lifestyle, and hormonal balance.

We explore the impact of specific nutrients on hormone production and regulation, offering insights into dietary choices that support women's endocrine health. From managing cortisol levels to promoting estrogen balance, the Metabolic Reset Diet provides a holistic framework for achieving and maintaining hormonal harmony.

Overcoming Plateaus and Setbacks

Women often encounter plateaus and setbacks in their wellness journeys, whether related to weight loss or overall metabolic health. This section offers guidance on navigating these challenges and leveraging the principles of the Metabolic Reset Diet to overcome obstacles.

We discuss the role of adaptation in metabolism, providing strategies to avoid plateaus and break through weight loss barriers. By understanding the body's responses to changes in diet and exercise, women can proactively adjust their approach to maintain progress and achieve their health goals.

Long-Term Metabolic Resilience

The ultimate desire for many women is not just short-term success but long-term metabolic resilience. This concluding part of the chapter reinforces the idea that the Metabolic Reset Diet is not a temporary solution but a sustainable lifestyle approach.

We explore how ongoing commitment to the principles of the diet can lead to lasting metabolic resilience. From adopting mindful eating habits to incorporating regular physical activity, women can cultivate a lifestyle that supports their metabolic health throughout different life stages.

In conclusion, this introductory chapter sets the stage for a transformative exploration of the Metabolic Reset Diet for Women. By understanding the foundations, overview, importance of metabolism, and addressing common concerns, readers gain insights into a holistic approach that goes beyond weight management, fostering overall well-being and vitality.

CHAPTER 1:
UNDERSTANDING METABOLISM

Embarking on the Metabolic Reset Diet journey necessitates a deep understanding of metabolism—the intricate biological process that serves as the body's engine. In this chapter, we unravel the complexities of metabolism, exploring its fundamental principles, the factors influencing it in women, and dispelling common misconceptions that might hinder the path to optimal health.

What Is Metabolism and How It Works: Decoding the Body's Engine

Metabolism is the dynamic and intricate set of chemical reactions that occur within the cells of the body to sustain life. It is the sum of all processes that convert food into energy, facilitating the maintenance and growth of cells, the regulation of body temperature, and the support of various physiological functions.

Breaking down metabolism into its two primary components provides clarity:

Anabolism: This involves the synthesis of complex molecules from simpler ones, such as building proteins from amino acids. It's the process of growth, repair, and the storage of energy.

Catabolism: This is the breakdown of complex molecules into simpler ones, releasing energy in the process. For instance, breaking down carbohydrates into glucose to provide energy for cellular activities.

The rate at which these processes occur collectively defines an individual's metabolic rate—the speed at which the body burns calories to maintain basic physiological functions during rest.

Understanding metabolism requires acknowledging the role of metabolic rate in determining how efficiently the body converts food into energy. This knowledge forms the foundation for the Metabolic Reset Diet, which aims to optimize metabolic efficiency through informed nutritional and lifestyle choices.

Factors that Influence Metabolism in Women: Navigating the Female Metabolic Landscape

Metabolism is not a one-size-fits-all concept, especially when it comes to women. Various factors contribute to the unique metabolic landscape of the female body, influencing how calories are burned, nutrients are processed, and energy is utilized. Here, we explore key factors shaping metabolism in women.

Hormonal Fluctuations:

Hormones play a pivotal role in regulating metabolism, and women experience cyclical hormonal changes throughout their lives. Menstruation, pregnancy, perimenopause, and menopause all bring about shifts in estrogen, progesterone, and other hormones, influencing metabolic rate and nutrient utilization.

Reproductive Stages:

Each reproductive stage brings its own metabolic considerations. For example, during pregnancy, the body's energy needs increase to support the growing fetus, while menopause introduces hormonal changes that may impact metabolism and body composition.

Genetic Predispositions:

Genetic factors contribute significantly to individual metabolic rates. Some women may inherit a naturally faster metabolism, while others may be more predisposed to weight gain. Understanding these genetic influences allows for personalized strategies within the Metabolic Reset Diet.

Body Composition:

The proportion of muscle to fat in the body directly impacts metabolism. Muscle tissue is metabolically active and burns more calories at rest than fat tissue. The Metabolic Reset Diet addresses strategies to support muscle preservation and development.

Dietary Choices:

The types of foods consumed, their nutrient composition, and meal timing influence metabolism. A diet rich in whole, nutrient-dense foods can enhance metabolic efficiency, while poor dietary choices may contribute to sluggish metabolism.

Physical Activity:

Regular exercise not only burns calories during the activity but also contributes to an elevated metabolic rate at rest. Incorporating both cardiovascular and strength training exercises is integral to the Metabolic Reset Diet for optimizing metabolism.

Impact of Age, Genetics, and Lifestyle on Metabolism

Understanding the influencers of metabolism provides a roadmap for women seeking to reset their metabolic health. Three primary influencers—age, genetics, and lifestyle—play pivotal roles in shaping metabolic efficiency.

Age and Metabolism:

Metabolism undergoes changes with age, and understanding these shifts is crucial for women navigating different life stages. In general, metabolism tends to slow down with age, primarily due to a natural loss of muscle mass. However, lifestyle factors and strategic dietary choices can mitigate age-related metabolic decline.

Genetics and Metabolic Variability:

Genetic predispositions contribute to individual differences in metabolism. Some women may inherently have a faster or slower metabolic rate, impacting their susceptibility to weight gain or difficulty losing weight. The Metabolic Reset Diet acknowledges these genetic influences, offering personalized approaches to optimize metabolic health.

Lifestyle Factors:

Lifestyle choices wield significant influence over metabolism. Factors such as diet, physical activity, stress management, and sleep directly impact metabolic rate. Adopting healthy habits within these lifestyle domains can positively influence metabolism, making it a focal point in the Metabolic Reset Diet.

By recognizing the interconnectedness of age, genetics, and lifestyle, women can empower themselves to make informed choices that support metabolic optimization. The Metabolic Reset Diet acts as a guide, tailoring strategies to individual needs and life stages.

Common Misconceptions About Metabolism: Dispelling Myths and Fostering Understanding

Misconceptions surrounding metabolism abound, often perpetuating confusion and hindering effective health management. In this section, we address and dispel common myths, fostering a clearer understanding of metabolism.

Myth: Metabolism Is Static:

One prevalent misconception is viewing metabolism as a fixed entity. Metabolism is dynamic and influenced by various factors. It adapts to changes in diet, physical activity, and other lifestyle factors. The Metabolic Reset Diet leverages this adaptability, emphasizing that metabolic health is within one's control.

Myth: Starvation Mode Slows Metabolism:

The idea that the body enters a "starvation mode" and slows metabolism in response to reduced calorie intake is a common myth. While prolonged extreme calorie restriction can impact metabolic rate, short-term fasting or controlled calorie reduction, as advocated by the Metabolic Reset Diet, can enhance metabolic efficiency.

Myth: All Calories Are Equal:

Not all calories are created equal, and this myth oversimplifies the relationship between calorie intake and metabolism. The source of calories—whether they come from nutrient-dense whole foods or processed, sugary items—plays a crucial role in influencing metabolic health. The Metabolic Reset Diet emphasizes the importance of quality, not just quantity, of calories.

Myth: Metabolism Slows Down After 40:

While it's true that metabolic rate tends to decline with age, the idea that it sharply plummets after turning 40 is a misconception. Strategic lifestyle choices, including proper nutrition and regular exercise, can mitigate age-related metabolic decline. The Metabolic Reset Diet provides tools to address and navigate these changes.

In dispelling these misconceptions, the Metabolic Reset Diet encourages women to approach metabolism with a nuanced understanding. By debunking myths and embracing accurate information, individuals can make informed choices that align with their health and wellness goals.

As we conclude this exploration of metabolism, women are equipped with the knowledge needed to navigate the intricate world of their body's engine. Understanding metabolism, acknowledging its influencers, and dispelling misconceptions lay the groundwork for the Metabolic Reset Diet's transformative journey. In the following chapters, we dive deeper into practical strategies, empowering women to optimize their metabolic health for sustainable well-being.

CHAPTER 2:
HORMONAL BALANCE AND METABOLISM

The interplay between hormones and metabolism is a symphony within the human body, orchestrating intricate processes that impact energy balance, weight management, and overall well-being. In this chapter, we delve into the profound connection between hormones and metabolism, exploring the significance of hormonal balance and its role in achieving optimal metabolic health.

The Connection Between Hormones and Metabolism: Harmonizing Body Functions

Hormones are chemical messengers produced by various glands in the endocrine system, influencing nearly every aspect of physiological function, including metabolism. The delicate dance between hormones and metabolism ensures that the body functions in a coordinated and balanced manner.

Insulin:

Insulin, produced by the pancreas, plays a central role in metabolism. It facilitates the uptake of glucose into cells for energy production and storage. Disruptions in insulin function, such as insulin resistance, can lead to metabolic issues and weight gain.

Thyroid Hormones:

Thyroid hormones, produced by the thyroid gland, regulate the body's metabolic rate. An imbalance in thyroid function can result in metabolic slowdown or acceleration, impacting energy expenditure and weight management.

Leptin and Ghrelin:

Leptin and ghrelin, often referred to as "hunger hormones," regulate appetite and satiety. Leptin signals fullness, while ghrelin stimulates hunger. Imbalances in these hormones can contribute to overeating and weight-related issues.

Cortisol:

Produced by the adrenal glands, cortisol is often associated with stress response. Chronic stress can lead to elevated cortisol levels, impacting metabolism and promoting fat storage, particularly in the abdominal area.

Understanding this intricate hormonal orchestra is fundamental to the Metabolic Reset Diet. It acknowledges that achieving optimal metabolism requires not only addressing nutritional and lifestyle factors but also fostering hormonal balance.

Hormonal Imbalances and their Impact on Weight Management

Hormonal imbalances can disrupt the harmonious relationship between hormones and metabolism, presenting challenges in weight management. Here, we explore how specific hormonal imbalances can impact the body's ability to regulate weight.

Insulin Resistance:

Insulin resistance occurs when cells become less responsive to insulin, leading to elevated blood sugar levels. This condition is often associated with weight gain, especially around the abdominal area, and can contribute to the development of type 2 diabetes.

Thyroid Disorders:

Hypothyroidism, characterized by an underactive thyroid, can slow down metabolism, leading to weight gain, fatigue, and other symptoms. Hyperthyroidism, on the other hand, can result in an overactive metabolism, causing unintended weight loss.

Leptin and Ghrelin Imbalance:

Dysregulation of leptin and ghrelin can disrupt appetite control. Leptin resistance, where the body doesn't respond adequately to leptin signals, can lead to overeating. Conversely, an imbalance that affects ghrelin may result in increased hunger and cravings.

Cortisol Dysregulation:

Chronic stress and elevated cortisol levels can contribute to weight gain, particularly around the midsection. This is often referred to as stress-induced or cortisol-induced obesity.

Recognizing the impact of these hormonal imbalances is crucial for women seeking to reset their metabolism. The Metabolic Reset Diet takes a holistic approach, incorporating strategies to address hormonal disruptions and restore balance.

Strategies to Support Hormonal Balance for Optimal Metabolism: Nurturing Hormonal Harmony

Achieving and maintaining hormonal balance is pivotal for optimizing metabolism. The Metabolic Reset Diet integrates a range of strategies designed to support hormonal harmony and promote metabolic health.

Balanced Nutrition:

Nutrient-dense, balanced meals play a central role in supporting hormonal balance. The diet emphasizes whole foods, rich in vitamins, minerals, and antioxidants, providing the essential building blocks for hormone production and regulation.

Strategic Macronutrient Intake:

Tailoring macronutrient intake—proteins, carbohydrates, and fats—supports specific hormonal functions. Adequate protein intake, for example, supports muscle preservation and hormone production, while healthy fats contribute to hormone synthesis.

Regular Physical Activity:

Exercise is a powerful tool for promoting hormonal balance. Both aerobic and strength-training exercises contribute to the regulation of insulin, cortisol, and other hormones. The Metabolic Reset Diet encourages a balanced and sustainable approach to physical activity.

Stress Management:

Chronic stress can disrupt hormonal balance, particularly cortisol regulation. Incorporating stress-management techniques such as mindfulness, meditation, or yoga is integral to the Metabolic Reset Diet.

Adequate Sleep:

Quality sleep is essential for hormonal health. Lack of sleep can impact insulin sensitivity, disrupt appetite-regulating hormones, and contribute to cortisol imbalances. The diet emphasizes the importance of prioritizing restorative sleep.

Limiting Processed Foods and Sugar:

Processed foods and excessive sugar intake can contribute to insulin resistance and disrupt hormonal balance. The Metabolic Reset Diet advocates for minimizing processed foods and adopting a low-sugar approach to support metabolic health.

By implementing these strategies, women can create an environment conducive to hormonal balance, fostering optimal metabolism and supporting their overall well-being.

Addressing Specific Hormonal Concerns (e.g., PCOS, Menopause)

Certain life stages and conditions, such as polycystic ovary syndrome (PCOS) and menopause, introduce unique hormonal considerations. The Metabolic Reset Diet recognizes the specific challenges associated with these concerns and provides tailored strategies.

Polycystic Ovary Syndrome (PCOS):

PCOS is a common hormonal disorder affecting women of reproductive age. It is characterized by imbalances in insulin, androgens (male hormones), and other hormones. The diet addresses PCOS by focusing on insulin regulation, supporting hormonal balance, and promoting weight management.

Menopause:

Menopause represents a significant hormonal transition, marked by a decline in estrogen and other hormonal fluctuations. The Metabolic Reset Diet acknowledges the impact of menopause on metabolism and offers strategies to support hormonal balance during this life stage. This includes dietary choices that alleviate symptoms and support overall well-being.

Recognizing the unique needs of women experiencing specific hormonal concerns allows the Metabolic Reset Diet to offer tailored guidance, ensuring that the strategies provided are not only effective but also mindful of individual health considerations.

As we conclude this exploration of hormonal balance and metabolism, women are armed with a comprehensive understanding of the intricate dance between hormones and metabolic health. The Metabolic Reset Diet serves as a guide, empowering women to nurture hormonal harmony, address imbalances, and achieve optimal metabolism. In the subsequent chapters, we delve into practical applications, offering actionable steps toward lasting metabolic mastery.

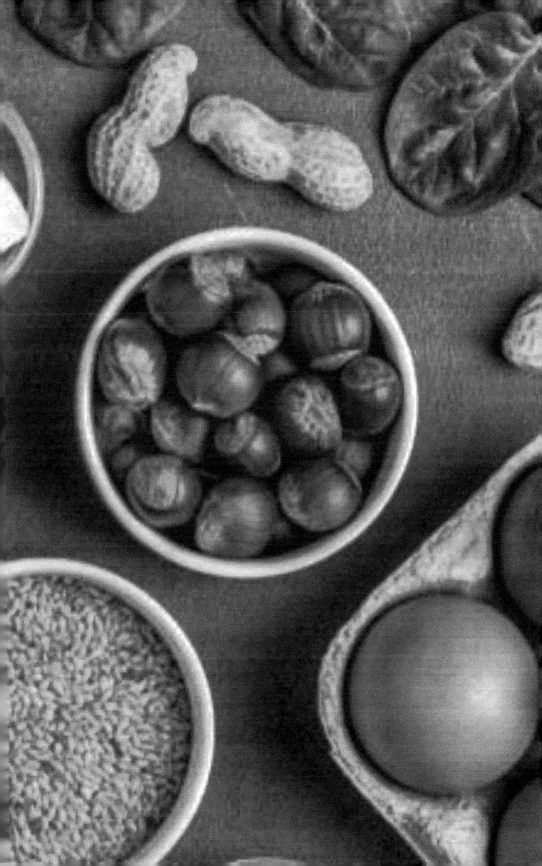

CHAPTER 3:
THE METABOLIC RESET DIET PRINCIPLES

As we delve into the core principles of the Metabolic Reset Diet, it is essential to grasp the overarching approach that sets the stage for metabolic transformation. This chapter provides an in-depth overview of the diet's principles, emphasizing a holistic and sustainable approach to optimize metabolism and foster lasting well-being.

Overview of the Metabolic Reset Diet Approach: A Holistic Blueprint for Wellness

The Metabolic Reset Diet is not a fleeting trend, but a comprehensive lifestyle approach designed to rejuvenate metabolism, promote sustainable weight management, and enhance overall well-being. At its core, the diet embraces the synergy between nutrition, lifestyle, and hormonal balance. Here's an overview of its key components:

Holistic Perspective:

The diet takes a holistic view, acknowledging that optimal metabolism is not solely about calories in and out. It considers the quality of nutrients, hormonal balance, and lifestyle factors, recognizing the interconnected nature of these elements.

Personalization:

One size does not fit all, and the Metabolic Reset Diet emphasizes personalization. It acknowledges the unique needs, preferences, and challenges of individuals, offering flexibility within a structured framework.

Sustainability:

Sustainability is a cornerstone of the diet. Rather than imposing drastic restrictions or short-term solutions, it promotes long-lasting changes that individuals can incorporate into their daily lives. This sustainability fosters ongoing metabolic health.

Focus on Health, Not Just Weight:

While weight management is a central goal, the diet goes beyond mere aesthetics. It places a strong emphasis on overall health, recognizing that a healthy body is not defined solely by its weight but by balanced hormones, energy levels, and a resilient metabolism.

Understanding this holistic and personalized approach is pivotal for individuals embarking on the Metabolic Reset Diet journey, setting the stage for comprehensive metabolic optimization.

Balancing Macronutrients for Metabolic Optimization

The Metabolic Reset Diet places a significant emphasis on the balance of macronutrients—proteins, carbohydrates, and fats—as a fundamental strategy for metabolic optimization. Achieving the right balance is crucial for supporting various physiological functions, hormonal balance, and energy production.

Proteins:

Proteins are the building blocks of the body, essential for muscle preservation, repair, and hormone production. The diet advocates for an adequate intake of lean proteins from sources such as poultry, fish, tofu, and legumes.

Carbohydrates:

Carbohydrates provide the body with energy, and their quality matters. The diet recommends complex carbohydrates, including whole grains, fruits, and vegetables, to ensure a sustained release of energy and support stable blood sugar levels.

Fats:

Healthy fats play a crucial role in hormone synthesis, brain function, and nutrient absorption. The diet encourages the consumption of sources like avocados, nuts, seeds, and olive oil, while limiting saturated and trans fats.

Strategic Meal Timing:

Beyond macronutrient balance, the diet recognizes the importance of strategic meal timing. Aligning nutrient intake with the body's natural circadian rhythms supports optimal metabolism and energy utilization throughout the day.

This balanced macronutrient approach serves as the foundation for the Metabolic Reset Diet, providing individuals with a sustainable and nourishing framework for metabolic health.

Understanding Calorie Intake and Expenditure

Calories are not merely units of energy but integral components of the metabolic equation. The Metabolic Reset Diet adopts a nuanced approach to calorie intake and expenditure, aiming for balance and sustainability.

Caloric Needs:

The diet begins by assessing individual caloric needs based on factors such as age, gender, activity level, and metabolic rate. This personalized approach ensures that individuals consume an appropriate amount of calories to support their unique requirements.

Caloric Balance:

Achieving a balance between calorie intake and expenditure is a central principle. While weight loss generally requires a caloric deficit, the diet emphasizes a gradual and sustainable approach, avoiding extreme restrictions that can negatively impact metabolism.

Metabolic Adaptation:

The diet recognizes the body's adaptive nature. As individuals progress, their metabolic needs may change. Adjustments to caloric intake are made mindfully, preventing the pitfalls of prolonged caloric restriction and supporting metabolic flexibility.

Quality Over Quantity:

The focus is not solely on caloric quantity but on the quality of calories consumed. Nutrient-dense foods are prioritized to ensure that caloric intake contributes to overall health and well-being.

By understanding the nuanced relationship between calories and metabolism, individuals following the Metabolic Reset Diet gain insights into a sustainable and health-focused approach to weight management.

Importance of Nutrient-Dense Foods and Portion Control: Crafting A Balanced Plate

Nutrient-dense foods and portion control are integral components of the Metabolic Reset Diet, contributing to both metabolic optimization and overall well-being.

Nutrient-Dense Foods:

The diet emphasizes the importance of choosing foods rich in essential nutrients—vitamins, minerals, antioxidants, and fiber. These foods not only support metabolic function but also provide the body with the tools it needs for optimal health.

Balanced Plate Approach:

Adopting a balanced plate approach involves incorporating a variety of foods from different food groups. This ensures a diverse nutrient intake and helps prevent nutrient deficiencies that can impact metabolism and overall health.

Portion Control:

Portion control is a key strategy for preventing overeating and promoting weight management. The diet encourages mindful eating, paying attention to hunger and fullness cues, and savoring each bite to avoid unnecessary caloric excess.

Hydration:

Adequate hydration is vital for metabolic function. The diet promotes regular water intake, recognizing that staying well-hydrated supports digestion, nutrient absorption, and overall metabolic efficiency.

This emphasis on nutrient-dense foods and portion control serves as a practical and accessible guide for individuals looking to cultivate a balanced and nourishing approach to their diet, aligning with the principles of the Metabolic Reset Diet.

As we conclude this exploration of the Metabolic Reset Diet principles, individuals are equipped with a comprehensive understanding of the approach that underpins metabolic optimization. This chapter serves as a guide for those seeking a sustainable, holistic, and personalized path to lasting well-being. In the subsequent chapters, we delve into practical applications, offering actionable steps toward achieving metabolic mastery and transformative health.

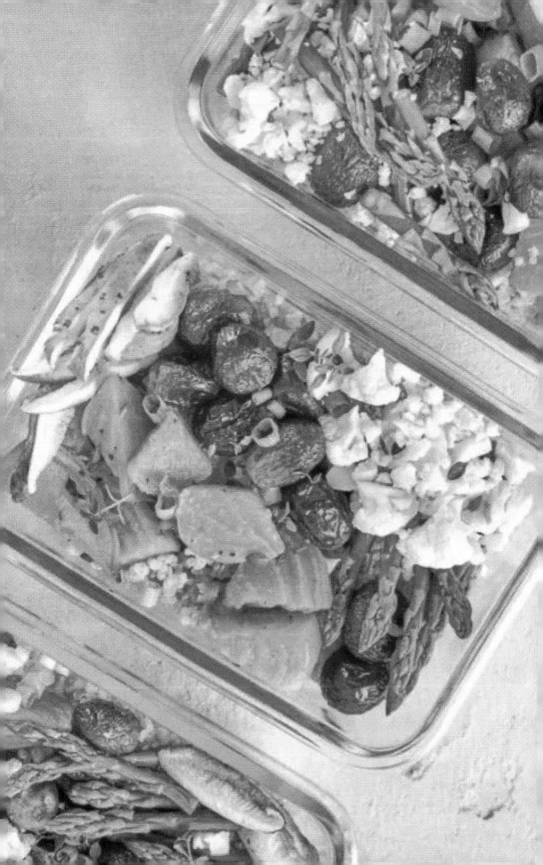

CHAPTER 4:
RESETTING YOUR METABOLISM: PHASE 1

Embarking on the Metabolic Reset Diet is a journey toward rejuvenating your metabolism and fostering lasting well-being. Phase 1 serves as the foundational step in this transformative process. This chapter introduces the initial phase, outlining its significance, specific guidelines, strategies for detoxification, and providing practical tools such as sample meal plans and recipes to guide individuals through this crucial stage of metabolic reset.

Phase 1 of the Metabolic Reset Diet marks the beginning of your journey toward metabolic rejuvenation. This initial phase sets the stage for sustainable changes by focusing on key principles:

Metabolic Priming:

The goal of Phase 1 is to prime your metabolism for optimal functioning. This involves creating an environment that supports hormonal balance, efficient energy utilization, and the elimination of toxins that may impede metabolic processes.

Transitioning to Nutrient-Dense Foods:

Phase 1 emphasizes the transition to nutrient-dense, whole foods that provide essential vitamins, minerals, and antioxidants. This shift lays the groundwork for sustained energy, hormonal harmony, and overall well-being.

Detoxification and Cleansing:

A key aspect of Phase 1 is to initiate the detoxification process, supporting the body's natural mechanisms for eliminating accumulated toxins. This not only aids metabolic function but also enhances overall health.

Meal Planning for Success:

Phase 1 introduces specific guidelines for meal planning, emphasizing a balanced intake of macronutrients, portion control, and strategic meal timing. These principles work synergistically to support your metabolic goals.

By understanding the overarching objectives of Phase 1, individuals can approach this stage with clarity and commitment, laying the foundation for transformative metabolic reset.

Specific Guidelines for Phase 1: Navigating Food Choices and Meal Planning

The success of Phase 1 hinges on adhering to specific guidelines tailored to optimize metabolism. These guidelines encompass food choices, meal planning strategies, and a mindful approach to nourishing your body.

Focus on Whole, Unprocessed Foods:

In Phase 1, prioritize whole, unprocessed foods that are rich in nutrients. Emphasize lean proteins, whole grains, fruits, vegetables, and healthy fats. Minimize or eliminate processed foods, sugary items, and excessive caffeine.

Balanced Macronutrient Intake:

Maintain a balanced intake of macronutrients, ensuring that each meal includes a combination of proteins, carbohydrates, and fats. This balance supports energy stability, hormone regulation, and metabolic efficiency.

Portion Control and Mindful Eating:

Practice portion control to prevent overeating and support weight management. Engage in mindful eating by paying attention to hunger and fullness cues, savoring each bite, and avoiding distractions during meals.

Strategic Meal Timing:

Implement strategic meal timing to align with natural circadian rhythms. Distribute your daily caloric intake across multiple meals, supporting sustained energy levels and preventing excessive calorie consumption in a single sitting.

Hydration as a Priority:

Prioritize hydration by drinking an adequate amount of water throughout the day. Staying well-hydrated supports metabolic processes, aids digestion, and contributes to overall well-being.

Following these guidelines during Phase 1 lays the groundwork for metabolic optimization, promoting a nutrient-rich and balanced approach to nourishment.

Strategies to Support Detoxification and Elimination of Toxins: Cleansing for Metabolic Clarity

Detoxification is a central focus of Phase 1, aiming to rid the body of accumulated toxins that may hinder metabolic function. The Metabolic Reset Diet employs specific strategies to support this cleansing process:

Hydration for Flush and Renewal:

Adequate water intake is a cornerstone of detoxification. Water helps flush out toxins through urine and supports various metabolic processes. Infuse your water with lemon or cucumber for added detox benefits.

Incorporate Detoxifying Foods:

Integrate foods known for their detoxifying properties into your meals. This includes cruciferous vegetables (broccoli, kale, cauliflower), berries rich in antioxidants, and herbs such as cilantro and parsley that support liver function.

Limit Exposure to Environmental Toxins:

Phase 1 encourages minimizing exposure to environmental toxins. This involves choosing organic produce, using natural cleaning products, and being mindful of potential sources of toxins in your environment.

Supportive Supplements:

Depending on individual needs, consider incorporating supportive supplements known for their detoxifying properties. This may include antioxidants like vitamin C or herbal supplements that aid liver function.

By embracing these detoxification strategies, individuals actively contribute to resetting their metabolism, promoting clarity, and laying the groundwork for sustained well-being.

Sample Meal Plans and Recipes for Phase 1: Practical Tools for Success

Implementing the guidelines of Phase 1 becomes more tangible with practical tools such as sample meal plans and recipes. These resources not only provide inspiration but also guide individuals in crafting balanced, nourishing meals aligned with the principles of the Metabolic Reset Diet.

14-Day Sample Meal Plan: Metabolic Reset Diet

I understand the importance of crafting a meal plan that not only supports metabolic reset but also provides nourishing and delicious meals to keep individuals motivated on their journey. This 14-day sample meal plan is designed to align with the principles of the Metabolic Reset Diet, emphasizing nutrient-dense foods, balanced macronutrients, portion control, and strategic meal timing.

Day 1:

Breakfast:

Quinoa Breakfast Bowl with Mixed Berries, Almonds, and a Drizzle of Honey

Lunch:

Grilled Chicken Salad with Mixed Greens, Cherry Tomatoes, Cucumber, and Balsamic Vinaigrette

Snack:

Greek Yogurt with Sliced Apple and a Sprinkle of Cinnamon

Dinner:

Baked Salmon with Quinoa and Roasted Vegetables (Broccoli, Carrots, Bell Peppers)

Day 2:

Breakfast:

Avocado Toast with Poached Egg and Tomato Slices

Lunch:

Lentil and Vegetable Soup with a Side of Whole Grain Crackers

Snack:

Fresh Fruit Salad (Strawberries, Pineapple, Kiwi)

Dinner:

Stir-Fried Tofu with Brown Rice and Steamed Broccoli

Day 3:

Breakfast:

Overnight Oats with Chia Seeds, Almond Milk, and Sliced Banana

Lunch:

Turkey and Hummus Wrap with Whole Wheat Tortilla, Spinach, and Bell Peppers

Snack:

Cottage Cheese with Mango Chunks

Dinner:

Grilled Shrimp Skewers with Quinoa and Grilled Asparagus

Day 4:

Breakfast:

Spinach and Feta Omelette with Whole Grain Toast

Lunch:

Quinoa Salad with Chickpeas, Cherry Tomatoes, Cucumber, and Lemon-Tahini Dressing

Snack:

Handful of Mixed Nuts (Almonds, Walnuts, Pistachios)

Dinner:

Baked Chicken Breast with Sweet Potato Mash and Steamed Green Beans

Day 5:

Breakfast:

Berry and Spinach Smoothie with Protein Powder and Almond Milk

Lunch:

Mediterranean Chickpea Salad with Feta Cheese and Kalamata Olives

Snack:

Sliced Pear with Almond Butter

Dinner:

Grilled Mahi-Mahi with Quinoa Pilaf and Roasted Brussels Sprouts

Day 6:

Breakfast:

Whole Grain Pancakes with Greek Yogurt and Fresh Berries

Lunch:

Caprese Salad with Sliced Avocado and Whole Grain Pita Bread

Snack:

Carrot Sticks with Hummus

Dinner:

Zucchini Noodles with Pesto Sauce and Grilled Chicken

Day 7:

Breakfast:

Smoked Salmon and Cream Cheese Bagel with Sliced Tomato and Red Onion

Lunch:

Turkey and Vegetable Stir-Fry with Brown Rice

Snack:

Orange Slices with a Sprinkle of Cinnamon

Dinner:

Beef and Vegetable Kebabs with Quinoa and Roasted Cauliflower

Day 8:

Breakfast:

Banana Walnut Muffins (Made with Whole Wheat Flour and Minimal Added Sugar)

Lunch:

Black Bean and Corn Salad with Avocado and Lime Dressing

Snack:

Yogurt Parfait with Granola and Mixed Berries

Dinner:

Grilled Portobello Mushrooms with Lentil Pilaf and Steamed Asparagus

Day 9:

Breakfast:

Oat Bran Porridge with Almond Milk, Sliced Peaches, and a Drizzle of Maple Syrup

Lunch:

Shrimp and Avocado Salad with Quinoa and Lemon-Herb Vinaigrette

Snack:

Apple Slices with a Thin Spread of Almond Butter

Dinner:

Baked Cod with Tomato and Olive Relish, Served with Couscous

Day 10:

Breakfast:

Greek Yogurt Smoothie Bowl with Mixed Berries, Granola, and Chia Seeds

Lunch:

Turkey and Vegetable Wrap with Whole Wheat Tortilla and Spinach

Snack:

Cottage Cheese with Pineapple Chunks

Dinner:

Grilled Tofu Skewers with Brown Rice and Stir-Fried Vegetables

Day 11:

Breakfast:

Scrambled Eggs with Spinach and Feta, Whole Grain Toast on the Side

Lunch:

Quinoa and Black Bean Bowl with Salsa, Guacamole, and Lime

Snack:

Handful of Trail Mix (Mix of Nuts, Seeds, and Dried Fruit)

Dinner:

Baked Chicken Thighs with Sweet Potato Wedges and Steamed Broccoli

Day 12:

Breakfast:

Whole Grain Waffles with Mixed Berry Compote and a Dollop of Greek Yogurt

Lunch:

Chickpea and Vegetable Curry with Basmati Rice

Snack:

Sliced Mango with Tajin Seasoning

Dinner:

Grilled Swordfish with Quinoa Salad and Grilled Zucchini

Day 13:

Breakfast:

Peanut Butter Banana Smoothie with Oats and Almond Milk

Lunch:

Tuna Salad Lettuce Wraps with Cherry Tomatoes and Cucumber

Snack:

Whole Grain Crackers with Hummus

Dinner:

Stir-Fried Beef with Broccoli and Brown Rice

Day 14:

Breakfast:

Veggie and Egg Breakfast Burrito with Whole Wheat Tortilla

Lunch:

Spinach and Quinoa Stuffed Bell Peppers with a Side of Greek Salad

Snack:

Kiwi and Strawberry Fruit Salad

Dinner:

Grilled Salmon with Lemon-Dill Sauce, Quinoa, and Steamed Asparagus

Note: This meal plan is a guide and may need adjustments based on individual dietary needs, preferences, and health conditions. Consultation with a healthcare professional or dietitian is recommended before starting any new diet plan.

Recipes for Phase 1:

Here are the 10 mouth-watering recipes designed for Phase 1 of the Metabolic Reset Diet, complete with ingredients, instructions, and nutritional information:

1. Grilled Chicken and Quinoa Salad with Lemon-Tahini Dressing:

Ingredients:

Grilled chicken breast slices

Quinoa

Mixed greens

Cherry tomatoes

Cucumber

Dressing: Lemon, tahini, olive oil, salt, and pepper.

Instructions:

Cook quinoa according to package instructions.

Grill chicken until fully cooked.

Assemble salad with mixed greens, quinoa, cherry tomatoes, cucumber, and grilled chicken.

Prepare dressing by whisking together lemon juice, tahini, olive oil, salt, and pepper.

Drizzle dressing over the salad.

Nutritional Information:

Protein: 25g

Carbohydrates: 30g

Fat: 15g

Fiber: 5g

Calories: 350

2. Detoxifying Green Smoothie Bowl:

Ingredients:

Spinach

Kale

Banana

Almond milk

Sliced strawberries

Chia seeds

Granola.

Instructions:

Blend spinach, kale, banana, and almond milk until smooth.

Pour into a bowl and top with sliced strawberries, chia seeds, and granola.

Nutritional Information:

Protein: 12g

Carbohydrates: 40g

Fat: 10g

Fiber: 8g

Calories: 280

3. Baked Salmon with Dill and Asparagus:

Ingredients:

Salmon fillets

Fresh dill

Garlic

Lemon

Asparagus

Olive oil

Salt and pepper.

Instructions:

Preheat oven to 375°F (190°C).

Season salmon with chopped dill, minced garlic, lemon juice, salt, and pepper.

Arrange salmon and asparagus on a baking sheet.

Bake for 15-20 minutes or until salmon is cooked through.

Nutritional Information:

Protein: 30g

Carbohydrates: 8g

Fat: 15g

Fiber: 3g

Calories: 320

4. Quinoa and Black Bean Stuffed Bell Peppers:

Ingredients:

Quinoa

Black beans

Corn

Spices (cumin, chili powder, paprika)

Bell peppers

Salsa.

Instructions:

Cook quinoa and mix with black beans, corn, and spices.

Cut bell peppers in half and remove seeds.

Stuff bell peppers with quinoa mixture.

Bake until peppers are tender.

Serve with a side of salsa.

Nutritional Information:

Protein: 15g

Carbohydrates: 35g

Fat: 5g

Fiber: 7g

Calories: 250

5. Lemon Garlic Shrimp Stir-Fry with Broccoli and Cauliflower Rice:

Ingredients:

Shrimp

Garlic

Lemon

Broccoli

Cauliflower rice

Soy sauce

Sesame oil.

Instructions:

Stir-fry shrimp with minced garlic, lemon juice, and a splash of soy sauce.

Add broccoli and continue to stir-fry until tender.

Serve over cauliflower rice.

Drizzle with sesame oil.

Nutritional Information:

Protein: 20g

Carbohydrates: 15g

Fat: 10g

Fiber: 5g

Calories: 220

6. Greek Yogurt Parfait with Berries and Almond Granola:

Ingredients:

Greek yogurt

Mixed berries (blueberries, raspberries, strawberries)

Almond granola

Honey (optional).

Instructions:

Layer Greek yogurt with mixed berries in a glass or bowl.

Sprinkle almond granola between the layers.

Drizzle with honey if desired.

Nutritional Information:

Protein: 18g

Carbohydrates: 30g

Fat: 8g

Fiber: 5g

Calories: 280

7. Avocado and Chickpea Lettuce Wraps:

Ingredients:

Ripe avocados

Chickpeas

Diced tomatoes

Cilantro

Lettuce leaves.

Instructions:

Mash avocados and chickpeas together.

Mix in diced tomatoes and chopped cilantro.

Spoon the mixture into lettuce leaves to create wraps.

Nutritional Information:

Protein: 10g

Carbohydrates: 20g

Fat: 15g

Fiber: 8g

Calories: 250

8. Zucchini Noodles with Pesto and Grilled Chicken:

Ingredients:

Zucchini

Homemade pesto

Grilled chicken breast

Cherry tomatoes.

Instructions:

Spiralize zucchini into noodles.

Toss with homemade pesto.

Top with grilled chicken slices and halved cherry tomatoes.

Nutritional Information:

Protein: 25g

Carbohydrates: 15g

Fat: 12g

Fiber: 5g

Calories: 300

9. Detoxifying Cucumber and Mint Infused Water:

Ingredients:

Cucumber slices

Fresh mint leaves

Water.

Instructions:

Combine cucumber slices and fresh mint in a pitcher of water.

Let it infuse in the refrigerator for at least an hour.

Nutritional Information:

No significant nutritional content.

10. Berry and Spinach Salad with Almond-Crusted Salmon:

Ingredients:

Salmon fillets with almond crust

Fresh spinach

Mixed berries

Almonds

Balsamic vinaigrette.

Instructions:

Coat salmon with almond crust and bake until golden.

Toss fresh spinach with mixed berries and sliced almonds.

Top with almond-crusted salmon.

Drizzle with balsamic vinaigrette.

Nutritional Information:

Protein: 28g

Carbohydrates: 18g

Fat: 20g

Fiber: 6g

Calories: 350

11. Grilled Lemon Herb Salmon:

Ingredients:

- 4 salmon fillets

- 2 tbsp fresh lemon juice

- 2 tbsp chopped fresh herbs (such as dill, parsley, or basil)

- 1 tbsp extra virgin olive oil

- Salt and pepper to taste

Instructions:

1. Preheat the grill to medium-high heat.

2. In a small bowl, combine lemon juice, chopped herbs, olive oil, salt, and pepper.

3. Brush the mixture over the salmon fillets, coating them evenly.

4. Place the salmon fillets on the grill and cook for about 4-5 minutes per side, or until cooked through.

5. Serve the grilled salmon with a side of steamed vegetables or a fresh salad.

Nutritional Information (approximate):

Calories: 300

Carbohydrates: 0g

Protein: 35g

Fat: 18g

Fiber: 0g

12. Detox Lentil Soup:

Ingredients:

- 1 cup dried green lentils, rinsed

- 1 onion, chopped

- 2 carrots, diced

- 2 celery stalks, diced

- 3 cloves garlic, minced

- 1 tsp turmeric

- 1 tsp cumin

- 6 cups vegetable broth

- 2 cups chopped kale

- Juice of 1 lemon

- Salt and pepper to taste

Instructions:

1. In a large pot, sauté the onion, carrots, celery, and garlic until softened.

2. Add the turmeric and cumin and cook for another minute.

3. Add the rinsed lentils and vegetable broth to the pot. Bring to a boil, then reduce heat and simmer for about 20-25 minutes, or until the lentils are tender.

4. Stir in the chopped kale and lemon juice. Cook for an additional 5 minutes.

5. Season with salt and pepper to taste.

6. Serve this comforting and detoxifying lentil soup hot.

Nutritional Information (approximate):

Calories: 250

Carbohydrates: 42g

Protein: 15g

Fat: 2g

Fiber: 15g

13. Baked Lemon Herb Chicken:

Ingredients:

- 4 boneless, skinless chicken breasts

- 2 tbsp fresh lemon juice

- 2 tbsp chopped fresh herbs (such as rosemary, thyme, or oregano)

- 2 cloves garlic, minced

- 1 tbsp extra virgin olive oil

- Salt and pepper to taste

Instructions:

1. Preheat the oven to 400°F (200°C).

2. In a small bowl, combine lemon juice, chopped herbs, minced garlic, olive oil, salt, and pepper.

3. Place the chicken breasts in a baking dish and pour the marinade over them, making sure to coat them evenly.

4. Bake in the preheated oven for about 20-25 minutes, or until the chicken is cooked through and no longer pink in the center.

5. Serve the baked lemon herb chicken with a side of steamed vegetables or a salad.

Nutritional Information (approximate):

Calories: 250

Carbohydrates: 2g

Protein: 40g

Fat: 8g

Fiber: 0g

14. Detoxifying Green Detoxifying Green Salad:

Ingredients:

- 4 cups mixed greens

- 1 cucumber, sliced

- 1 avocado, diced

- ¼ cup sliced almonds

- 2 tbsp chopped fresh cilantro

- Juice of 1 lime

- 1 tbsp extra virgin olive oil

- Salt and pepper to taste

Instructions:

1. In a large bowl, combine mixed greens, cucumber slices, diced avocado, sliced almonds, and chopped cilantro.

2. In a small bowl, whisk together lime juice, olive oil, salt, and pepper.

3. Drizzle the dressing over the salad and toss to combine.

4. Serve this refreshing and detoxifying green salad as a side or add grilled chicken or salmon for a complete meal.

Nutritional Information (approximate):

Calories: 300

Carbohydrates: 16g

Protein: 7g

Fat: 25g

Fiber: 9g

15. Detoxifying Turmeric Ginger Smoothie:

Ingredients:

- 1 cup unsweetened almond milk

- 1 frozen banana

- 1-inch piece of fresh ginger, peeled and grated

- 1 tsp ground turmeric

- 1 tbsp chia seeds

- 1 tbsp honey or maple syrup (optional for sweetness)

- Ice cubes (optional)

Instructions:

1. In a blender, combine almond milk, frozen banana, grated ginger, ground turmeric, chia seeds, and honey or maple syrup.

2. Blend until smooth and creamy.

3. Add ice cubes if desired and blend again.

4. Pour into a glass and enjoy this detoxifying and immune-boosting smoothie.

Nutritional Information (approximate):

Calories: 200

Carbohydrates: 40g

Protein: 4g

Fat: 5g

Fiber: 7g

16. Sweet Potato and Kale Hash with Poached Eggs:

Ingredients:

Sweet potatoes, diced

Kale, chopped

Poached eggs

Olive oil

Garlic, minced

Paprika, salt, and pepper.

Instructions:

Sauté diced sweet potatoes in olive oil until golden.

Add minced garlic and chopped kale.

Season with paprika, salt, and pepper.

Serve with poached eggs on top.

Nutritional Information:

Protein: 15g

Carbohydrates: 30g

Fat: 10g

Fiber: 7g

Calories: 280

17. Cauliflower and Broccoli Detox Soup:

Ingredients:

Cauliflower, chopped

Broccoli, chopped

Vegetable broth

Onion, diced

Turmeric, cumin, salt, and pepper.

Instructions:

Sauté diced onion until translucent.

Add chopped cauliflower and broccoli.

Pour in vegetable broth and season with turmeric, cumin, salt, and pepper.

Simmer until vegetables are tender.

Nutritional Information:

Protein: 10g

Carbohydrates: 20g

Fat: 5g

Fiber: 8g

Calories: 180

18. Quinoa and Vegetable Stir-Fry:

Ingredients:

Quinoa

Mixed vegetables (bell peppers, snap peas, carrots)

Tofu, cubed

Soy sauce

Sesame oil

Ginger, minced.

Instructions:

Cook quinoa according to package instructions.

Stir-fry tofu and mixed vegetables in sesame oil.

Add cooked quinoa and soy sauce.

Finish with minced ginger.

Nutritional Information:

Protein: 18g

Carbohydrates: 35g

Fat: 10g

Fiber: 6g

Calories: 320

19. Turmeric and Garlic Baked Chicken Thighs:

Ingredients:

Chicken thighs

Turmeric

Garlic powder

Lemon juice

Olive oil

Rosemary, chopped.

Instructions:

Coat chicken thighs with turmeric, garlic powder, and lemon juice.

Drizzle with olive oil and sprinkle with chopped rosemary.

Bake until golden and cooked through.

Nutritional Information:

Protein: 25g

Carbohydrates: 1g

Fat: 15g

Fiber: 0g

Calories: 280

20. Chia Seed Pudding with Mixed Berries:

Ingredients:

Chia seeds

Almond milk

Mixed berries (blueberries, strawberries, raspberries)

Maple syrup.

Instructions:

Mix chia seeds with almond milk and let it sit overnight.

Layer chia pudding with mixed berries.

Drizzle with a touch of maple syrup.

Nutritional Information:

Protein: 10g

Carbohydrates: 25g

Fat: 8g

Fiber: 12g

Calories: 230

As we conclude the exploration of Phase 1 of the Metabolic Reset Diet, individuals are equipped with a comprehensive understanding of its significance, specific guidelines, detoxification strategies, and practical tools. Phase 1 serves as the launchpad for metabolic transformation, setting the stage for sustained well-being and optimized metabolism. In the subsequent chapters, we delve into further phases, providing a roadmap for continued success on your journey toward metabolic mastery.

CHAPTER 5:
RESETTING YOUR METABOLISM: PHASE 2

Transitioning from Phase 1 to Phase 2 of the Metabolic Reset Diet

As you progress from Phase 1 to Phase 2 of the Metabolic Reset Diet, it's essential to understand the nuanced changes that accompany this transition. Phase 1 primarily focuses on jumpstarting your metabolism, eliminating toxins, and establishing a foundation for healthy eating habits. Phase 2 builds upon this foundation, introducing subtle adjustments to further optimize your metabolic reset journey.

One key aspect of the transition is the continuation of nutrient-dense, whole foods that support your body's nutritional needs. However, in Phase 2, there is a gradual reintroduction of certain food groups that were limited in Phase 1. This might include healthy carbohydrates like sweet potatoes or whole grains, providing additional energy sources while maintaining the principles of balanced nutrition.

Moreover, Phase 2 encourages a heightened awareness of portion control. While Phase 1 establishes the groundwork for mindful eating, Phase 2 refines this practice. Portion control plays a pivotal role in maintaining a balanced calorie intake, preventing overconsumption, and supporting sustainable weight management.

The transition also involves evaluating how your body responds to different foods. In Phase 2, you could reintroduce certain foods systematically, observing how they impact your energy levels, digestion, and overall well-being. This self-awareness allows for a more personalized approach to your metabolic reset, emphasizing foods that work optimally for your unique physiology.

Adjusting Macronutrient Ratios and Calorie Intake

Phase 2 of the Metabolic Reset Diet introduces a more nuanced approach to macronutrient ratios and calorie intake. While Phase 1 establishes a baseline, Phase 2 allows for personalized adjustments based on individual needs, goals, and responses to specific food groups.

Balanced Macronutrient Ratios: In Phase 2, the emphasis remains on a balanced distribution of macronutrients—proteins, carbohydrates, and fats. However, individuals may find their bodies respond differently to various ratios. Some may thrive with a slightly higher carbohydrate intake, while others may benefit from a more moderate approach. Fine-tuning macronutrient ratios ensures that your dietary plan aligns with your metabolic goals and supports sustainable energy levels.

Calorie Intake Optimization: While Phase 1 often involves a controlled calorie intake to kickstart metabolism, Phase 2 allows for a more tailored approach. Depending on factors such as activity level, metabolic rate, and individual goals, adjustments to calorie intake may be necessary. This phase encourages a flexible yet mindful approach to calorie consumption, ensuring that energy needs are met without unnecessary surplus.

The key is to approach these adjustments with a holistic understanding of your body's signals. Regular monitoring of energy levels, mood, and overall well-being provides valuable insights into whether your current macronutrient ratios and calorie intake are supporting your metabolic reset effectively.

Incorporating Exercise and Physical Activity for Metabolic Enhancement

Physical activity is a crucial component of Phase 2 in the Metabolic Reset Diet. While Phase 1 focuses on dietary changes, Phase 2 introduces a strategic approach to exercise that synergizes with your nutritional goals. The combination of targeted exercises and increased physical activity contributes significantly to metabolic enhancement and overall well-being.

Strategic Exercise Selection: Phase 2 introduces a variety of exercises that complement your metabolic reset journey. Strength training, cardiovascular exercises, and flexibility workouts are incorporated strategically based on individual fitness levels and preferences. Strength training plays a pivotal role in building lean muscle mass, which can positively impact your basal metabolic rate.

Consistent Physical Activity: Beyond structured workouts, Phase 2 encourages consistent physical activity throughout the day. This includes non-exercise activities like walking, taking the stairs, or engaging in recreational activities. Consistent movement contributes to calorie expenditure, supports overall cardiovascular health, and reinforces the metabolic benefits initiated in Phase 1.

Mindful Movement Practices: In addition to traditional exercises, Phase 2 introduces mindful movement practices such as yoga or tai chi. These practices not only enhance physical flexibility and balance but also promote stress reduction. Stress management is crucial for metabolic health and incorporating mindful movement aids in achieving a holistic approach to well-being.

Sample Meal Plans and Recipes for Phase 2

Creating a sustainable and enjoyable dietary plan is essential in Phase 2 of the Metabolic Reset Diet. This phase builds upon the foundational principles of Phase 1, incorporating a broader range of nutrient-dense foods while maintaining a focus on balanced nutrition. Below are sample meal plans and recipes tailored for Phase 2:

Sample Meal Plan:

Day 1:

Breakfast:

Scrambled Eggs with Spinach and Feta

Whole Grain Toast

Lunch:

Quinoa Salad with Roasted Vegetables and Grilled Chicken

Snack:

Greek Yogurt with Berries

Dinner:

Baked Cod with Lemon-Dill Sauce

Steamed Broccoli

Sweet Potato Mash

Day 2:

Breakfast:

Vegetable omelet with spinach, bell peppers, and mushrooms cooked in olive oil.

Snack:

Greek yogurt with mixed berries.

Lunch:

Grilled chicken breast with roasted vegetables (such as broccoli, cauliflower, and carrots).

Snack:

Celery sticks with almond butter.

Dinner:

Baked salmon with quinoa and steamed asparagus.

Dessert:

Mixed fruit salad.

Day 3:

Breakfast:

Overnight oats made with rolled oats, almond milk, chia seeds, and topped with sliced banana and a sprinkle of cinnamon.

Snack:

Hard-boiled egg and carrot sticks.

Lunch:

Quinoa and black bean salad with mixed greens, cherry tomatoes, and avocado.

Snack:

Apple slices with almond butter.

Dinner:

Grilled turkey breast with roasted Brussels sprouts and sweet potatoes.

Dessert:

Dark chocolate squares.

Day 4:

Breakfast:

Green smoothie made with spinach, frozen berries, almond milk, and a scoop of protein powder.

Snack:

Greek yogurt with sliced almonds and a drizzle of honey.

Lunch:

Lentil soup with a side of mixed greens and lemon-tahini dressing.

Snack:

Celery sticks with hummus.

Dinner:

Baked cod with quinoa and steamed broccoli.

Dessert:

Chia seed pudding with coconut milk and fresh berries.

Day 5:

Breakfast:

Veggie scramble with eggs, bell peppers, onions, and mushrooms.

Snack:

Cottage cheese with pineapple chunks.

Lunch:

Grilled chicken Caesar salad with romaine lettuce, cherry tomatoes, and homemade Caesar dressing.

Snack:

Carrot sticks with guacamole.

Dinner:

Stir-fried tofu with mixed vegetables and brown rice.

Dessert:

Sliced mango.

Day 6:

Breakfast:

Protein pancakes made with mashed bananas, oats, and protein powder, topped with mixed berries.

Snack:

Hard-boiled egg and cucumber slices.

Lunch:

Quinoa-stuffed bell peppers with a side of mixed greens.

Snack:

Mixed nuts and seeds.

Dinner:

Grilled shrimp skewers with roasted zucchini and quinoa.

Dessert:

Baked apple slices with cinnamon.

Day7:

Breakfast:

Veggie omelet with spinach, tomatoes, and feta cheese.

Snack:

Greek yogurt with sliced almonds and a drizzle of honey.

Lunch:

Lentil and vegetable stir-fry with brown rice.

Snack:

Apple slices with almond butter.

Dinner:

Baked chicken breast with roasted Brussels sprouts and quinoa.

Dessert:

Dark chocolate squares.

Day 7:

Breakfast:

Green smoothie made with kale, pineapple, almond milk, and a scoop of protein powder.

Snack:

Cottage cheese with mixed berries.

Lunch:

Grilled salmon with quinoa and steamed asparagus.

Snack:

Carrot sticks with hummus.

Dinner:

Turkey meatballs with zucchini noodles and marinara sauce.

Dessert:

Chia seed pudding with coconut milk and sliced almonds.

Day 9:

Breakfast:

Overnight oats made with rolled oats, almond milk, chia seeds, and topped with sliced banana and a sprinkle of cinnamon.

Snack:

Hard-boiled egg and cucumber slices.

Lunch:

Quinoa and black bean salad with mixed greens, cherry tomatoes, and avocado.

Snack:

Mixed nuts and seeds.

Dinner:

Baked cod with roasted Brussels sprouts and sweet potatoes.

Dessert:

Sliced mango.

Day 10:

Breakfast:

Veggie scramble with eggs, bell peppers, onions, and mushrooms.

Snack:

Greek yogurt with mixed berries.

Lunch:

Lentil soup with a side of mixed greens and lemon-tahini dressing.

Snack:

Apple slices with almond butter.

Dinner:

Stir-fried tofu with mixed vegetables and brown rice.

Dessert:

Baked apple slices with cinnamon.

Day 11:

Breakfast:

Protein pancakes made with mashed bananas, oats, and protein powder, topped with mixed berries.

Snack:

Hard-boiled egg and carrot sticks.

Lunch:

Grilled chicken Caesar salad with romaine lettuce, cherry tomatoes, and homemade Caesar dressing.

Snack:

Celery sticks with hummus.

Dinner:

Baked salmon with quinoa and steamed broccoli.

Dessert:

Mixed fruit salad.

Day 12:

Breakfast:

Green smoothie made with spinach, frozen berries, almond milk, and a scoop of protein powder.

Snack:

Greek yogurt with sliced almonds and a drizzle of honey.

Lunch:

Lentil and vegetable stir-fry with brown rice.

Snack:

Mixed nuts and seeds.

Dinner:

Grilled shrimp skewers with roasted zucchini and quinoa.

Dessert:

Dark chocolate squares.

Day 13:

Breakfast:

Veggie omelet with spinach, tomatoes, and feta cheese.

Snack:

Cottage cheese with pineapple chunks.

Lunch:

Quinoa-stuffed bell peppers with a side of mixed greens.

Snack:

Apple slices with almond butter.

Dinner:

Turkey meatballs with zucchini noodles and marinara sauce.

Dessert:

Chia seed pudding with coconut milk and fresh berries.

Day 14:

Breakfast:

Overnight oats made with rolled oats, almond milk, chia seeds, and topped with sliced banana and a sprinkle of cinnamon.

Snack:

Hard-boiled egg and cucumber slices.

Lunch:

Quinoa and black bean salad with mixed greens, cherry tomatoes, and avocado.

Snack:

Carrot sticks with hummus.

Dinner:

Baked chicken breast with roasted Brussels sprouts and quinoa.

Dessert:

Sliced mango.

Remember to adjust portion sizes and ingredients according to your specific dietary needs and consult with a healthcare professional before starting any new diet plan.

Recipes For Phase 2

Quinoa Salad with Roasted Vegetables and Grilled Chicken

Ingredients:

Quinoa

Mixed Vegetables (bell peppers, zucchini, cherry tomatoes)

Olive Oil

Lemon Juice

Grilled Chicken Breast

Feta Cheese

Fresh Herbs (parsley, mint)

Instructions:

Cook quinoa according to package instructions.

Toss mixed vegetables in olive oil and roast until tender.

Combine quinoa, roasted vegetables, and grilled chicken slices.

Drizzle with lemon juice, sprinkle feta cheese and fresh herbs.

Nutritional Information:

Protein: 25g

Carbohydrates: 40g

Fat: 10g

Fiber: 8g / Calories: 350

Turkey and Avocado Wrap

Ingredients:

Sliced Turkey Breast

Avocado

Leafy Greens (lettuce, spinach)

Whole Wheat Tortilla

Instructions:

Lay out the whole wheat tortilla.

Add sliced turkey, avocado, and leafy greens.

Roll the ingredients into a wrap.

Nutritional Information:

Protein: 20g

Carbohydrates: 30g

Fat: 15g

Fiber: 6g / Calories: 300

1. Grilled Salmon and Quinoa Power Bowl:

Ingredients:

Grilled salmon fillet

Cooked quinoa

Roasted sweet potatoes

Steamed broccoli

Avocado slices

Lemon-tahini dressing.

Instructions:

Arrange quinoa in a bowl, top with grilled salmon.

Add roasted sweet potatoes, steamed broccoli, and avocado slices.

Drizzle with lemon-tahini dressing.

Nutritional Information:

Protein: 30g

Carbohydrates: 40g

Fat: 15g

Fiber: 10g

Calories: 400

2. Mediterranean Chickpea and Vegetable Stir-Fry:

Ingredients:

Chickpeas

Mixed vegetables (bell peppers, cherry tomatoes, spinach)

Olive oil

Garlic and herbs.

Instructions:

Sauté chickpeas and mixed vegetables in olive oil.

Season with garlic and your favorite Mediterranean herbs.

Nutritional Information:

Protein: 15g

Carbohydrates: 30g

Fat: 8g

Fiber: 9g

Calories: 280

3. Quinoa and Kale Stuffed Bell Peppers:

Ingredients:

Quinoa

Chopped kale

Black beans

Diced tomatoes

Spices (cumin, chili powder)

Bell peppers.

Instructions:

Cook quinoa and mix with kale, black beans, diced tomatoes, and spices.

Stuff bell peppers with the quinoa mixture.

Nutritional Information:

Protein: 18g

Carbohydrates: 35g

Fat: 5g

Fiber: 8g / Calories: 320

4. Lemon Herb Chicken with Asparagus and Brown Rice:

Ingredients:

Grilled chicken breast

Asparagus spears

Brown rice

Lemon

Fresh herbs (rosemary, thyme).

Instructions:

Grill chicken with lemon and fresh herbs.

Roast asparagus in olive oil.

Serve over cooked brown rice.

Nutritional Information:

Protein: 25g

Carbohydrates: 40g

Fat: 10g

Fiber: 6g

Calories: 380

5. Spinach and Feta Turkey Burgers:

Ingredients:

Ground turkey

Chopped spinach

Feta cheese

Whole wheat burger buns.

Instructions:

Mix ground turkey with chopped spinach and crumbled feta.

Shape into patties and grill.

Serve on whole wheat burger buns.

Nutritional Information:

Protein: 20g

Carbohydrates: 30g

Fat: 15g

Fiber: 5g

Calories: 320

6. Roasted Vegetable and Quinoa Salad:

Ingredients:

Roasted vegetables (zucchini, cherry tomatoes, bell peppers)

Quinoa

Mixed greens

Balsamic vinaigrette.

Instructions:

Toss roasted vegetables with cooked quinoa and mixed greens.

Drizzle with balsamic vinaigrette.

Nutritional Information:

Protein: 15g

Carbohydrates: 35g

Fat: 8g

Fiber: 7g

Calories: 300

7. Tofu and Vegetable Coconut Curry:

Ingredients:

Firm tofu

Mixed vegetables (broccoli, carrots, bell peppers)

Coconut milk

Curry paste.

Instructions:

Sauté tofu and mixed vegetables in a pan.

Add coconut milk and curry paste for a flavorful curry.

Nutritional Information:

Protein: 18g

Carbohydrates: 25g

Fat: 12g

Fiber: 6g

Calories: 320

8. Shrimp and Vegetable Stir-Fry with Cauliflower Rice:

Ingredients:

Shrimp

Mixed vegetables (snap peas, carrots, bell peppers)

Cauliflower rice

Soy sauce.

Instructions:

Stir-fry shrimp and mixed vegetables in soy sauce.

Serve over cauliflower rice.

Nutritional Information:

Protein: 22g

Carbohydrates: 15g

Fat: 10g

Fiber: 5g

Calories: 280

9. Avocado and Quinoa Stuffed Portobello Mushrooms:

Ingredients:

Portobello mushrooms

Quinoa

Avocado

Cherry tomatoes

Balsamic glaze.

Instructions:

Roast portobello mushrooms in the oven.

Fill with a mixture of cooked quinoa, diced avocado, and cherry tomatoes.

Drizzle with balsamic glaze.

Nutritional Information:

Protein: 12g

Carbohydrates: 30g

Fat: 10g

Fiber: 8g

Calories: 280

10. Teriyaki Chicken and Broccoli Brown Rice Bowl:

Ingredients:

Teriyaki chicken

Steamed broccoli

Brown rice

Sesame seeds.

Instructions:

Cook teriyaki chicken and steam broccoli.

Serve over a bed of brown rice.

Sprinkle with sesame seeds for added crunch.

Nutritional Information:

Protein: 28g

Carbohydrates: 45g

Fat: 8g

Fiber: 7g

Calories: 380

These sample meal plans and recipes showcase the variety and flexibility available in Phase 2 of the Metabolic Reset Diet. The emphasis on nutrient-dense foods, balanced macronutrients, and strategic exercise positions you for continued metabolic enhancement and overall well-being.

11. Veggie Egg Muffins:

Ingredients:

6 eggs

1/2 cup mixed vegetables (such as spinach, bell peppers, and onions), chopped

1/4 cup feta cheese, crumbled

Salt and pepper to taste

Instructions:

1. Preheat oven to 375°F (190°C).

2. In a bowl, whisk together eggs, mixed vegetables, feta cheese, salt, and pepper.

3. Grease a muffin tin with cooking spray or line with paper liners.

4. Pour the egg mixture evenly into the muffin cups.

5. Bake for 20-25 minutes or until the egg muffins are set and lightly golden on top.

6. Allow them to cool slightly before removing from the muffin tin.

7. Serve as a protein-packed breakfast or snack.

Nutritional Information (per serving - 2 egg muffins):

- Calories: 180

- Protein: 14g

- Fat: 12g

- Carbohydrates: 3g

- Fiber: 1g

12. Greek Yogurt Parfait:

Ingredients:

1 cup Greek yogurt

1/4 cup mixed berries (such as blueberries, strawberries, and raspberries)

2 tablespoons granola

1 tablespoon honey (optional)

Instructions:

1. In a glass or bowl, layer Greek yogurt, mixed berries, and granola.

2. Drizzle with honey if desired.

3. Repeat the layers.

4. Serve as a nutritious and satisfying breakfast or dessert.

Nutritional Information (per serving):

- Calories: 220

- Protein: 20g

- Fat: 5g

- Carbohydrates: 25g

- Fiber: 3g

13. Baked Salmon with Lemon-Dill Sauce:

Ingredients:

4 salmon fillets

Juice of 1 lemon

2 tablespoons fresh dill, chopped

1 tablespoon olive oil

Salt and pepper to taste

Instructions:

1. Preheat oven to 400°F (200°C).

2. Place salmon fillets on a baking sheet lined with parchment paper.

3. In a small bowl, mix lemon juice, fresh dill, olive oil, salt, and pepper.

4. Brush the lemon-dill mixture over the salmon fillets.

5. Bake for 12-15 minutes or until the salmon is cooked through and flakes easily with a fork.

6. Serve with steamed asparagus or roasted vegetables.

Nutritional Information (per serving):

Calories: 300

Protein: 30g

Fat: 18g

Carbohydrates: 1g

Fiber: 0g

14. Turkey and Vegetable Stir-Fry:

Ingredients:

1 lb ground turkey

2 cups mixed vegetables (such as bell peppers, broccoli, and snap peas)

2 cloves garlic, minced

2 tablespoons low-sodium soy sauce

1 tablespoon sesame oil

1 teaspoon ginger, grated

Salt and pepper to taste

Instructions:

1. Heat sesame oil in a large skillet or wok over medium heat.

2. Add ground turkey and cook until browned, breaking it up into small pieces.

3. Add minced garlic, grated ginger, and mixed vegetables to the skillet. Stir-fry for 5-7 minutes or until vegetables are tender.

4. Stir in soy sauce, salt, and pepper. Cook for an additional 2 minutes.

5. Serve over cauliflower rice or quinoa.

Nutritional Information (per serving):

- Calories: 280

- Protein: 26g

- Fat: 15g

- Carbohydrates: 12g

- Fiber: 4g

15. Grilled Lemon Herb Chicken:

Ingredients:

4 boneless, skinless chicken breasts

Juice of 2 lemons

2 tablespoons olive oil

2 garlic cloves, minced

1 tablespoon fresh thyme leaves

Salt and pepper to taste

Instructions:

1. In a bowl, combine lemon juice, olive oil, minced garlic, thyme leaves, salt, and pepper.

2. Place chicken breasts in a shallow dish and pour the marinade over them. Let marinate for at least 30 minutes.

3. Preheat grill to medium-high heat. Grill chicken for 6-8 minutes per side or until cooked through.

4. Serve with steamed vegetables or a side salad.

Nutritional Information (per serving):

- Calories: 250

- Protein: 30g

- Fat: 12g

- Carbohydrates: 2g

- Fiber: 0g

16. Baked Cod with Roasted Vegetables:

Ingredients:

4 cod fillets

2 tablespoons lemon juice

2 tablespoons olive oil

1 teaspoon dried dill

Salt and pepper to taste

2 cups mixed vegetables (such as broccoli, bell peppers, and carrots)

Instructions:

1. Preheat oven to 400°F (200°C).

2. In a small bowl, mix lemon juice, olive oil, dried dill, salt, and pepper.

3. Place cod fillets in a baking dish and brush with the lemon-dill mixture. Let marinate for 10 minutes.

4. Arrange mixed vegetables around the cod fillets and drizzle with olive oil. Season with salt and pepper.

5. Bake for 15-20 minutes or until the fish is cooked through and the vegetables are tender.

6. Serve with a side of quinoa or brown rice.

Nutritional Information (per serving):

- Calories: 220

- Protein: 30g

- Fat: 8g

- Carbohydrates: 10g

- Fiber: 4g

17. Quinoa and Black Bean Salad:

Ingredients:

1 cup cooked quinoa

1 cup canned black beans, rinsed and drained

1 cup cherry tomatoes, halved

1 small cucumber, diced

1/4 cup red onion, finely chopped

2 tablespoons fresh cilantro, chopped

Juice of 1 lime

1 tablespoon olive oil

Salt and pepper to taste

Instructions:

1. In a large bowl, combine cooked quinoa, black beans, cherry tomatoes, cucumber, red onion, and cilantro.

2. In a small bowl, whisk together lime juice, olive oil, salt, and pepper.

3. Pour the dressing over the quinoa mixture and toss to combine.

4. Refrigerate for at least 30 minutes before serving to allow the flavors to meld.

5. Serve as a light lunch or side dish.

Nutritional Information (per serving):

- Calories: 180

- Protein: 7g

- Fat: 5g

- Carbohydrates: 29g

Phase 2 of the Metabolic Reset Diet represents a dynamic shift from the initial stages, emphasizing individualization and optimization. The transition involves fine-tuning your dietary approach, adjusting macronutrient ratios, and incorporating targeted exercises for comprehensive metabolic enhancement. With a focus on sustainable practices and a diverse array of nutrient-dense foods, Phase 2 sets the stage for continued success on your metabolic reset journey. It's a phase of empowerment, allowing you to harness the knowledge gained in Phase 1 and apply it to create a personalized, effective, and enjoyable approach to resetting your metabolism.

CHAPTER 6:
MAINTAINING A HEALTHY METABOLISM

Strategies for Long-Term Sustainability and Maintenance

Achieving a metabolic reset is a commendable accomplishment, but the real measure of success lies in sustaining these positive changes over the long term. Here are strategic approaches to ensure the continued health of your metabolism:

1. Consistent Nutritional Habits:

Maintaining a healthy metabolism starts with consistent nutritional habits. Transition from the structured phases of your metabolic reset to a balanced, sustainable eating pattern. Emphasize whole foods, lean proteins, and a variety of colorful vegetables. Avoid extreme diets and focus on a well-rounded approach that meets your nutritional needs.

2. Regular Physical Activity:

Exercise isn't just a means to an end; it's a lifelong commitment to your overall health and metabolic well-being. Incorporate a mix of cardiovascular exercises, strength training, and flexibility workouts into your routine. Find activities you enjoy making exercise a sustainable part of your lifestyle. Consistency is key for maintaining a healthy metabolism.

3. Adequate Hydration:

Staying well-hydrated is often underestimated in its impact on metabolism. Water plays a crucial role in various metabolic processes, including digestion and nutrient transport. Make hydration a habit by carrying a reusable water bottle and setting reminders to drink throughout the day.

4. Sufficient Sleep:

Quality sleep is a non-negotiable component of maintaining a healthy metabolism. Lack of sleep can disrupt hormonal balance, leading to increased cravings and a sluggish metabolism. Aim for 7-9 hours of quality sleep per night. Establish a relaxing bedtime routine and create a conducive sleep environment for sustained metabolic health.

Building Healthy Habits and A Balanced Lifestyle

Creating and maintaining healthy habits is foundational to sustaining a well-functioning metabolism. Here's how to build habits that contribute to a balanced lifestyle:

1. Meal Planning and Preparation:

Plan your meals ahead of time to avoid impulsive, unhealthy choices. Dedicate time each week for meal preparation, ensuring that nutritious options are readily available. This habit not only supports your metabolism but also saves time and promotes mindful eating.

2. Mindful Eating Practices:

Cultivate mindful eating habits to enhance your relationship with food. Pay attention to hunger and fullness cues, savor the flavors of your meals, and minimize distractions during eating. Mindful eating fosters a healthy connection with food, reducing the likelihood of overeating and supporting metabolic balance.

3. Regular Health Check-Ups:

Regular health check-ups are essential for monitoring your metabolic health. Schedule routine visits with healthcare professionals to assess key indicators such as blood pressure, cholesterol levels, and blood sugar. Early detection of any deviations allows for prompt intervention and ensures sustained metabolic well-being.

4. Stay Active Throughout the Day:

In addition to structured workouts, prioritize staying active throughout the day. Break up long periods of sitting with short walks, take the stairs, and engage in activities you enjoy. These simple yet consistent movements contribute to overall metabolic health and prevent stagnation.

Tips for Overcoming Plateaus and Challenges

Plateaus and challenges are inevitable on any wellness journey. Knowing how to navigate them is crucial for maintaining a healthy metabolism. Here are tips for overcoming obstacles:

1. Periodic Dietary Adjustments:

As your body adapts to changes, periodic dietary adjustments can prevent plateaus. Consider rotating different food sources, adjusting macronutrient ratios, or incorporating intermittent fasting. These variations keep your metabolism responsive and promote ongoing progress.

2. Revise Exercise Routine:

Plateaus in physical activity often lead to metabolic stagnation. Periodically revise your exercise routine by introducing new activities, increasing intensity, or changing workout formats. This prevents your body from adapting too efficiently and ensures continuous metabolic challenges.

3. Manage Stress Effectively:

Chronic stress can impede metabolic function. Develop stress-management strategies such as meditation, deep breathing exercises, or engaging in hobbies. Prioritize self-care to mitigate the impact of stress on your metabolism and overall well-being.

4. Consult with Professionals:

If you encounter persistent challenges, seeking professional guidance is a wise step. Consult with a registered dietitian, fitness trainer, or healthcare provider to assess your individual circumstances. They can provide personalized recommendations to overcome hurdles and keep your metabolism on track.

Mindset and Motivation for Sustained Success

Maintaining a healthy metabolism is not just about physical habits; it's also deeply tied to mindset and motivation. Cultivate a positive mental framework to sustain your success:

1. Set Realistic Goals:

Establish realistic, achievable goals that align with your long-term vision. Unrealistic expectations can lead to frustration and undermine motivation. Celebrate small victories along the way and recognize that sustainable changes take time.

2. Embrace Progress, Not Perfection:

Understand that perfection is unattainable, and setbacks are a natural part of the journey. Instead of focusing on perfection, celebrate your progress. Learn from challenges, adapt, and continue moving forward with a resilient mindset.

3. Foster Intrinsic Motivation:

Find intrinsic motivation by connecting with the deeper reasons behind your wellness journey. Whether it's improved energy, better health, or enhanced overall well-being, cultivating internal motivations strengthens your commitment for the long haul.

4. Build a Support System:

Surround yourself with a supportive community. Share your goals with friends, family, or a fitness group. Having a support system provides encouragement during challenging times and reinforces your commitment to maintaining a healthy metabolism.

5. Educate Yourself Continuously:

Stay informed about the latest research and information related to metabolic health. Continuous education empowers you to make informed choices, adapt your strategies, and evolve with the ever-changing landscape of wellness.

Maintaining a healthy metabolism is a holistic endeavor that requires a combination of consistent habits, resilience in the face of challenges, and a positive mindset. By incorporating these strategies for long-term sustainability, building healthy habits, overcoming plateaus, and fostering a resilient mindset, you set the stage for sustained success on your metabolic health journey. Remember, it's not just about reaching a destination; it's about embracing a lifestyle that supports your well-being for years to come.

CHAPTER 7:
BEYOND THE DIET: SUPPORTING OVERALL HEALTH

Importance of Holistic Health Beyond Just Metabolism

While metabolic health is a crucial aspect of overall well-being, it is essential to recognize the broader importance of holistic health. Beyond metabolism, holistic health encompasses various interconnected elements that contribute to a woman's overall vitality and longevity.

1. Emotional Well-Being:

Holistic health involves nurturing emotional well-being. Stress, anxiety, and other emotional factors can significantly impact metabolism. Practices such as mindfulness meditation, journaling, and seeking emotional support play a pivotal role in maintaining a healthy balance between the mind and body.

2. Social Connections:

Human beings are inherently social creatures, and fostering meaningful connections contributes to holistic health. Engaging in positive social interactions, building a support system, and cultivating strong relationships can positively influence mental and emotional well-being, indirectly benefiting metabolic health.

3. Spiritual Wellness:

For many, spiritual wellness is an integral component of holistic health. This may involve connecting with one's beliefs, practicing gratitude, or engaging in activities that bring a sense of purpose. A holistic approach recognizes the importance of aligning physical health with spiritual and emotional fulfillment.

4. Environmental Factors:

The environment we live in can impact our health. From the air we breathe to the quality of water we consume, considering environmental factors is crucial. A holistic approach includes promoting a clean and sustainable environment, recognizing its role in supporting overall health.

Addressing Digestive Health and Gut Microbiome

1. The Gut-Metabolism Connection:

A growing body of research highlights the intricate connection between gut health and metabolism. The gut microbiome, a complex community of microorganisms in the digestive tract, influences various metabolic processes. Maintaining a balanced and diverse gut microbiome is essential for optimal metabolism.

2. Importance of Fiber-Rich Foods:

Fiber is a key player in promoting digestive health. It aids in regular bowel movements, supports the growth of beneficial gut bacteria, and helps control blood sugar levels. Including a variety of fiber-rich foods such as fruits, vegetables, and whole grains is crucial for a healthy gut and, consequently, a well-functioning metabolism.

3. Probiotics and Fermented Foods:

Probiotics, often found in fermented foods like yogurt, kefir, and sauerkraut, introduce beneficial bacteria to the gut. These microorganisms contribute to a balanced gut microbiome, enhancing digestion and absorption of nutrients. Including probiotic-rich foods supports digestive health and can positively impact metabolism.

4. Hydration for Digestive Well-Being:

Proper hydration is fundamental to digestive health. Water helps break down food, aids in the absorption of nutrients, and supports the overall functioning of the digestive system. Adequate water intake contributes to regular bowel movements, preventing issues such as constipation.

Managing Stress and Sleep for Optimal Metabolism

1. The Impact of Stress on Metabolism:

Chronic stress can disrupt hormonal balance and negatively impact metabolism. Stress hormones, such as cortisol, can influence appetite, cravings, and the storage of fat. Managing stress through effective coping mechanisms is vital for maintaining optimal metabolic function.

2. Stress-Reducing Practices:

Incorporating stress-reducing practices into daily life is essential for overall well-being. Techniques such as yoga, meditation, deep breathing exercises, and progressive muscle relaxation can help alleviate stress. Regular practice of these techniques contributes to a more balanced and resilient metabolism.

3. Importance of Quality Sleep:

Quality sleep is a cornerstone of holistic health, directly influencing metabolic processes. During sleep, the body undergoes crucial repair and restoration. Lack of sleep can disrupt hormonal balance, increase appetite, and impair glucose metabolism. Establishing consistent sleep patterns supports overall metabolic health.

4. Creating a Sleep-Optimized Environment:

Creating a sleep-friendly environment is key to improving sleep quality. This involves maintaining a comfortable room temperature, minimizing noise and light, and establishing a calming pre-sleep routine. Prioritizing sleep hygiene contributes to better rest and supports metabolic well-being.

Supplements and Additional Support for Women's Health

1. Essential Nutrients for Women:

Women have unique nutritional needs, particularly during various life stages such as pregnancy, lactation, and menopause. Essential nutrients like calcium, vitamin D, iron, and folate are crucial for women's health. Depending on individual requirements, supplementation may be recommended to ensure optimal nutrient intake.

2. Omega-3 Fatty Acids:

Omega-3 fatty acids play a vital role in supporting cardiovascular health, cognitive function, and inflammatory response. These essential fats are found in fatty fish, flaxseeds, and walnuts. Supplements, such as fish oil capsules, can be considered to ensure an adequate intake of omega-3s.

3. Probiotic Supplements:

While fermented foods contribute to a healthy gut, some individuals may benefit from probiotic supplements. These supplements provide concentrated doses of beneficial bacteria, supporting digestive health and the gut microbiome. Consulting with a healthcare professional can help determine the appropriate probiotic supplementation.

4. Adaptogenic Herbs for Stress Management:

Adaptogenic herbs like ashwagandha and rhodiola are known for their stress-relieving properties. These herbs help the body adapt to stressors and promote overall resilience. Incorporating adaptogens, whether through supplements or teas, can be a valuable addition to stress management strategies.

In conclusion, the journey towards optimal health goes beyond a singular focus on metabolism. Holistic well-being encompasses emotional, social, and spiritual aspects, acknowledging the interconnectedness of these elements. Addressing digestive health, managing stress, prioritizing quality sleep, and considering additional support through supplements contribute to a comprehensive approach to women's health. By recognizing and nurturing these various facets, individuals can embark on a transformative journey towards sustained overall well-being. Remember, true health is a harmonious blend of physical, mental, and emotional vitality.

CONCLUSION:

Recap of Key Concepts and Takeaways from the Metabolic Reset Diet

As we conclude this journey through the Metabolic Reset Diet for Women, it's essential to recap the key concepts and takeaways that form the foundation of this transformative approach to health.

1. Understanding Metabolism:

The journey began with a deep dive into metabolism—the intricate process by which our bodies convert food into energy. We explored how factors such as age, genetics, and lifestyle influence metabolism, debunking common misconceptions along the way. Armed with this knowledge, readers gained a comprehensive understanding of their body's metabolic intricacies.

2. Hormonal Balance and Metabolism:

Chapter 2 delved into the critical connection between hormones and metabolism. We explored how hormonal imbalances, whether related to conditions like PCOS or menopause, can impact weight management. The chapter provided practical strategies to support hormonal balance, empowering readers to optimize their metabolic health through informed choices.

3. The Metabolic Reset Diet Principles:

Central to this journey is the Metabolic Reset Diet itself. In Chapter 3, readers gained insights into the principles guiding this transformative approach. From the importance of balancing macronutrients to understanding calorie intake and the significance of nutrient-dense foods, the chapter laid the groundwork for implementing practical and sustainable dietary changes.

4. Resetting Your Metabolism: Phase 1:

Chapter 4 introduced the initial phase of the Metabolic Reset Diet. Readers received detailed guidelines on food choices, meal planning, and strategies to support detoxification. Sample meal plans and recipes provided practical examples, making the transition into Phase 1 accessible and enjoyable.

5. Resetting Your Metabolism: Phase 2:

Moving into Phase 2, Chapter 5 guided readers through the transition and adjustment process. Adjusting macronutrient ratios, incorporating exercise, and embracing new sample meal plans and recipes marked a progressive step in the metabolic reset journey.

6. Maintaining a Healthy Metabolism:

Chapter 6 focused on the long-term sustainability of the metabolic reset. Readers learned strategies for building healthy habits, overcoming plateaus, and nurturing a mindset conducive to sustained success. By embracing consistency, regular health check-ups, and staying active, readers fortified their commitment to maintaining a healthy metabolism.

7. Beyond the Diet: Supporting Overall Health:

Expanding the perspective, Chapter 7 explored holistic health beyond just metabolism. Addressing digestive health and the gut microbiome, managing stress, and considering supplements for women's health enriched the understanding of how interconnected elements contribute to overall vitality.

Encouragement and Motivation for Readers to Embark on their Metabolic Reset Journey

Embarking on a metabolic reset journey is a profound commitment to one's well-being. As we conclude, let's draw inspiration from the progress made and find the motivation to continue this transformative path.

1. Celebrating Progress:

Reflect on the journey thus far. Celebrate the progress, both big and small. Whether you've embraced new dietary habits, incorporated regular exercise, or experienced positive shifts in energy and mood, each step is a testament to your commitment to a healthier, more vibrant life.

2. Embracing Resilience:

The metabolic reset journey is not without its challenges, and resilience is key. If you've encountered setbacks or faced unexpected hurdles, remember that resilience is not about avoiding difficulties but about bouncing back stronger. Embrace challenges as opportunities for growth and learning.

3. Cultivating Mindfulness:

Mindful awareness is a powerful tool on this journey. Pay attention to how your body responds to dietary changes, exercise, and lifestyle adjustments. Cultivating mindfulness enhances your connection with your body, making it easier to identify what supports your unique metabolic needs.

4. Setting Realistic Goals:

In the pursuit of optimal health, set realistic and sustainable goals. Understand that transformations take time, and the journey is as important as the destination. Setting achievable goals ensures that progress is steady and enjoyable.

Conclusion

As we close this chapter, remember that the metabolic reset journey is ongoing. It's a dynamic process of self-discovery, growth, and sustained well-being. By applying the principles learned, embracing resilience, and exploring additional resources, you empower yourself to navigate this journey with wisdom and confidence. Your commitment to optimal health is a gift to yourself—embrace it with enthusiasm, and may your journey be filled with continued success and vitality.

Printed in Great Britain
by Amazon

d336657f-0a1b-4faa-88c1-b65975632fb5R01